Advanced Technologies in Healthcare

Shuli Guo · Lina Han · Yanan Guo

Advanced Technologies in Healthcare

AI, Signal Processing, Digital Twins and 5G

Springer

Shuli Guo
National Key Lab of Autonomous Intelligent Unmanned Systems
School of Automation
Beijing Institute of Technology
Beijing, China

Yanan Guo
National Key Lab of Autonomous Intelligent Unmanned Systems
School of Automation
Beijing Institute of Technology
Beijing, China

Lina Han
Department of Cardiology
The Second Medical Center, National Clinical Research Center for Geriatric Diseases
Chinese PLA General Hospital
Beijing, China

ISBN 978-981-99-9584-4 ISBN 978-981-99-9585-1 (eBook)
https://doi.org/10.1007/978-981-99-9585-1

This Springer imprint is published by the registered company Springer Nature Singapore Pte Ltd.
The registered company address is: 152 Beach Road, #21-01/04 Gateway East, Singapore 189721, Singapore

Paper in this product is recyclable.

We warmly celebrate Hainan College of Software Technology for the 100th birthday.

Preface

Professor Lina Han and I have been committed ourselves to the research of artificial intelligence medicine for more than 20 years. Using mathematics, communication, automation, medicine and other technologies, we studied physiological signals, including ECG, EEG, heart sound, oxygen saturation, respiration and other remote accurate and rapid acquisition and transmission. We also investigated the precise identification and positioning of 14 kinds of human behaviors including walking, running, turning inside and outside the room. We probed the artificial intelligence applications in medical images, including noise removal, feature extraction, reconstruction, etc. There are 3 published national standards and 36 authorized patents for our applications in the field of medical field. At the same time, our presented technologies already break through some bottlenecks in the domestic and international medical engineering forefronts.

During the process of theoretical research and application practices, we found that blockchain, digital twin technology, cloud, fog and edge computing technology of 5G communication are important technologies to promote the future advancement of intelligent medicine. This book presents the latest advances of the above technologies, their medical applications, medical image processing and disease management as follows. Chapter 1 presents the common AI algorithms of machine learning and deep learning, their main applications such as medical diagnostics and drug discoveries, especially the challenges in the healthcare. Chapter 2 lists the core technologies such as blockchain, the blockchain-based AI system and some applications in the intelligent sharing of electronic medical records and the traceability of drugs. Chapter 3 introduces some models of medical imaging and their factors of the image quality. Chapter 4 introduces the status and prospects of digital twin technology in the field of healthcare. Chapter 5 introduces the frameworks of cloud, fog and edge computing and their applications in the healthcare. Finally, many innovative standards of smart medicine devices are presented.

This book provides some technological information for graduate students and engineers in the fields of medicine, software engineering, automation and computer science, and at the same time, it offers some ideas and methods to medical engineering research and applications.

Beijing, China Shuli Guo
May 2023

Acknowledgements

We wish to thank many professors who have given us comments concerning these topics in this book and those friends who have encouraged us to carry it out over the years. It is difficult to do anything in life without the friends' help, and many of my friends have contributed much to this book.

Our sincere gratitude goes especially to Academician of the Chinese Academy of Sciences, Prof. Huang Lin of Peking University; Academician of the Chinese Academy of Engineering, Prof. Chen Jie of China Education Department; and Academician of the Chinese Academy of Engineering, Prof. Fu Mengyin of Nanjing University of Science and Technology, Prof. Irene Moroz of Oxford University, Prof. Wang Long of Peking University, Prof. Cao Xiankun of Education Department of Hainan Province, Prof. Ren Fujun of China Association for Science and Technology, Prof. Fan Li, Prof. He Kunlun, Director Li Tianzhi, Director Li Xingjie, Prof. Wang Chunxi, Prof. Luo Leiming, Prof. Sheng Li, Prof. Cao Feng of Chinese PLA General Hospital, Prof. Ma Wanbiao of University of Science and Technology Beijing, Prof. Wang Junzheng, Prof. Wu Qinghe, Prof. Xia Yuanqing, Prof. Wang Zhaohua, Prof. Zhang Baihai, Prof. Liu Xiangdong of Beijing Institute of Technology.

We wish to thank our colleagues and friends Prof. Chen Huiyang, Prof. Liu Mingpeng, Prof. He Jinxu, Prof. Fu Chuanyi and Prof. Wang Qingmin, Prof. Luo Xiaoyou, Prof. Liu laiquan, Prof. Huang Hao, Prof. Ma Jie and Prof. Fu Tian of Hainan College of Software Technology.

We wish to thank our graduate Ph.D. degree students Song Xiaowei, Wang Guowei, Wang Hui, Wu Lei, Zhao Zhilei, Wu Yue, Cekderi Anil Baris and Jia Jiaoyu and our graduate master's degree students Li Qiuyue, Zhang Yating, Yan Biyu, Chao Yue, Huang Haichun and Xue Jianing.

We wish to thank Hainan Province Science and Technology Special Fund under the Grant ZDYF2021GXJS205 and Hainan College of Software Technology.

We also wish to take this opportunity to thank Dr. Huang Shuting of Dalian University of Technology for critically reviewing the entire manuscript and giving constructive comments on our manuscript.

We are truly indebted to Mr. Wayne Hu for working with me for 5 months to take care of the typing and preparation of this book's manuscript. Lastly, this book is dedicated to Mr. Niraja Deshmukh, Mrs. Nobuko Kamikawa and their colleagues for their active efforts.

Beijing, China
May 2023

Shuli Guo
Lina Han
Yanan Guo

Contents

About the Authors

Prof. Shuli Guo was born in 1973 in Inner Mongolia, P. R. China. He received his bachelor's degree (1995), master's degree (1998) from Inner Mongolia Normal University and his Ph.D. degree from Peking University (2001). Dr. Guo worked as a postdoctoral researcher from January 2002 to April 2004 at Tsinghua University, as a researcher fellow from January 2008 to September 2008 at Akita Prefectural University and as a postdoctoral researcher from September 2008 to September 2009 at Oxford University. Prof. Guo's research interests include classical control theory and application, medical image processing, medical data analysis, typical chronic disease analysis and remote medical monitoring. Recently, he has published nearly 70 impactful paper, 4 monographs, 34 authorized Chinese patents and 15 authorized software copyrights. He has published 3 Chinese national standards and handed in 9 Chinese national standards/industrial standards for approval. He obtained one third prize for military medical achievements, one third prize of science and technology of the Chinese Medical Association and one third prize of Beijing Medical Science and Technology. And he is the member of Chinese national technical committee for professional standardization (2021–2026), the head of China geriatric disease standardized diagnosis and treatment society of CAGG (2018–2023) and the chief expert of Chinese national key research and development program (2017–2021).

Prof. Lina Han was born in 1973 in Jilin Province, P. R. China. She received her Med. bachelor's degree (1995), Med. master's degree (2000) and Ph.D. degree (2003) from Jilin University. Dr. Han worked as a postdoctoral researcher from July 2003 to April 2005 at Chinese PLA General Hospital and as a research fellow from August 2008 to September 2009 at Kyoto University. And now, she works as a research fellow at the Department of Cardiovascular Internal Medicine, National Clinical Research Center for Geriatric Diseases, the 2rd Medicine Centre of Chinese PLA General Hospital and Chinese PLA Medical School. Her research interests focus on many 3D modeling problems on cardiovascular systems and their medical solutions.

Ms. Yanan Guo was born in 2000 in Shandong Province, P. R. China. She received her bachelor's degree (2021) from Shandong University. Now she is a master's degree postgraduate in Beijing Institute of Technology. Her main research interests are the area of application of AI technology in healthcare.

Chapter 1
Artificial Intelligence Technology

1.1 Introduction

Britannica defines AI as "The ability of a digital computer or computer-controlled robot to perform tasks commonly associated with intelligent beings", which can be termed as a science of training systems in order to emulate human work with automation and learning. The machine can ingest a large amount of data information, extract their main features, determine the way of analysis and edit codes to execute the computation and production of intelligent outputs.

AI is fully used to accomplish tasks that, in the past, might have been only done by human beings themselves. In the past three decades, AI has been widely utilized in many disciplines, especially in medicine, and has achieved the following accomplishments.

- Prediction. It involves getting long- and short-term variability in the data to forecast the likelihood of illness.
- Image recognition. It determines if the observed nodes on a CT scan are benign or malignant.
- Classification. It evaluates the patients' electrocardiograms (ECG) and then classifies them to support the subsequent disease diagnosis according to their beating data.
- Pattern recognition. For example, it automatically analyzes of the semantic content of lung cancer and uses color slice image data for its early diagnosis.
- Speech text. It transcribes the agents' voice messages into the text to detect sentiments and other evaluations.
- Natural language processing. It summarizes and analyzes large document collections, then generates the diagnosis reports and makes future predictions with the help of software.

The following primary technologies such as deep learning, machine learning and neural networks are the foundation stones to gain complete comprehension of AI

S. Guo et al., *Advanced Technologies in Healthcare*,
https://doi.org/10.1007/978-981-99-9585-1_1

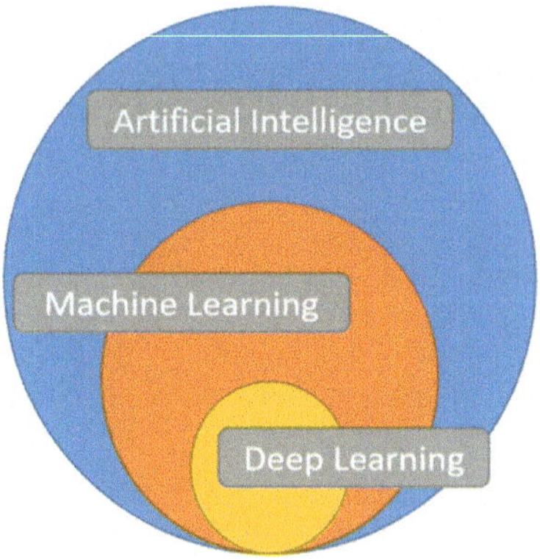

Fig. 1.1 Difference among AI, machine learning and deep learning in the digital world

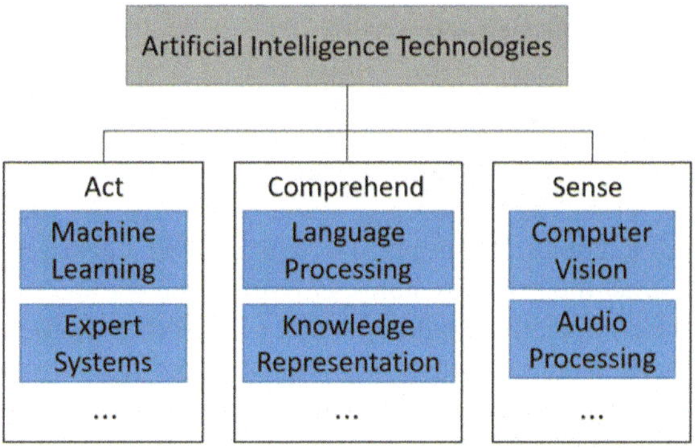

Fig. 1.2 Defining AI and machine learning

itself and its derivatives. Figure 1.1 depicts a schematic diagram of the difference among AI, machine learning and deep learning concepts. In most cases, machine learning is a subset of AI (Fig. 1.2 shows different scopes between AI and machine learning). Deep learning is generally termed as a machine learning technique, which is functioned using neural networks.

1.2 Machine Learning

1.2.1 Introduction

In 1959, Arthur Samuel used the phrase "Machine Learning". It is a very basic type to parse data with algorithms, learn and make predictions. Machine learning algorithms develop a mathematical model on sample data as the training set to reach predictions or decisions, which is hardly programmed to carry out the task. Machine learning is highly dependent on the observed data, which is the main source. The main purpose is to allow machines or computers to learn and improve subsequent actions without human involvements or helps.

1.2.2 Methods

The machine learning algorithms are mainly classified into supervised learning, unsupervised learning, semi-supervised learning and reinforced learning.

For supervised learning, their algorithms can predict future events through learning past information, which start from the selection of a good training dataset, and output an inferred function for the predictions. The above system can sustainably offer targets for a new input after training, compare their output with the intended output and finally decrease the errors to correct the model. The common supervised learning algorithms are as follows:

- Decision Tree. The decision tree algorithm uses a tree structure to establish a decision model based on the attributes of the data, which is often used to solve classification problems.
- Naive Bayes. The naive Bayes algorithm is based on the Bayes probability theory, which is called naive because it assumes that each input variable is independent. The algorithm is mainly composed of two stages: firstly, the probabilities under different conditions are calculated respectively through classifying the experimental samples, then the probability of different conditions is calculated and compared so as to complete the test sample classification when the test sample is input.
- Support Vector Machine. The support vector machine algorithm distinguishes two data groups in the n-dimensional space by constructing a (n-1)-dimensional separated hyperplane, which transforms the input data into a high-dimensional space, generates an n-dimensional vector and maximizes the margin between the two data groups to optimally separate different categories. Support vector machine model is shown as Fig. 1.3.

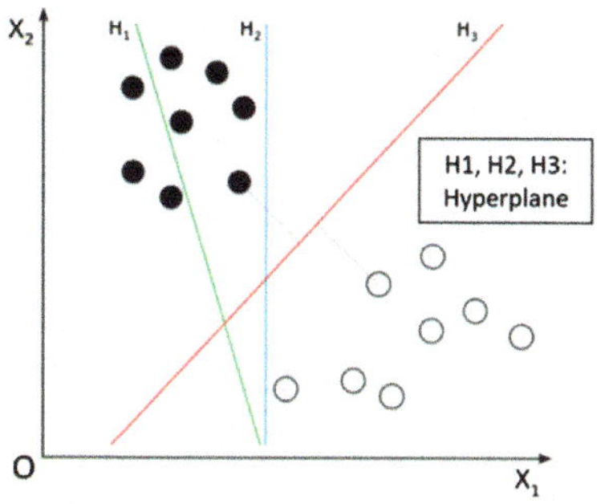

Fig. 1.3 Support vector machine model

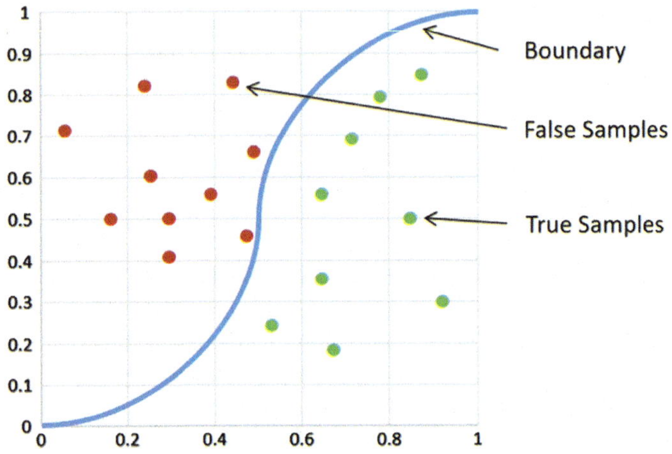

Fig. 1.4 Logistic regression model

- Logistic Regression. The logistic regression algorithm is to predict the probability of an event by fitting a logistic function, which is generally composed of three steps. First, a suitable prediction function is constructed and generally defined by the h function, which is used to predict the results of the input data. Then, a loss function is constructed to represent the deviation between the predicted output and the training data. The "loss" of all training data, which is called as the J function, is comprehensively considered through their sum or average and represents the deviation of the predicted value of all training data from the actual. Finally, the minimum value of the J function is found by generally using the gradient descent method. The model of logistic regression is shown as Fig. 1.4.

For the unsupervised learning, the used information doesn't need to label or classify and simultaneously the machine does not have fixed data sets. It tests the given datasets, draws some inferences from them to describe their hidden structures and proposes the correspond solutions to interpret the above data by using the binary logic mechanism. The common unsupervised learning algorithms are as follows:

- Singular Value Decomposition. The Eq. (1.1) denotes the singular value decomposition. In actual, the least dimensional nonzero singular values are tried to select, and the obtained matrix can be restored to represent the main features of the given datasets, which can be shown as (1.2),

$$M_{m\times n} = U_{m\times m}\sum\nolimits_{m\times n} V^T_{n\times n} \tag{1.1}$$

$$M_{m\times n} \approx U_{m\times r}\sum\nolimits_{r\times r} V^T_{r\times n} \tag{1.2}$$

where M is a matrix of $m \times n$, U is a matrix of $m \times m$, $\sum$ is a matrix of $m \times n$ in which every element on the diagonal is singular value and others are 0, and

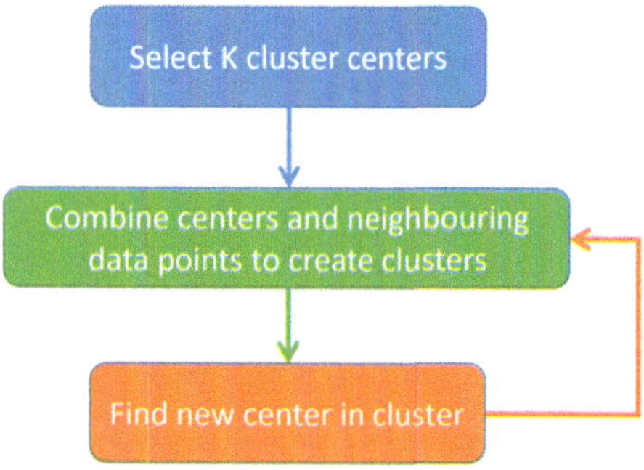

Fig. 1.5 Flowchart of *K*-means algorithm

V is a matrix of $n \times n$. U and V are both unitary matrices, that is, they satisfy $U^T U = I$, $V^T V = I$.

- Apriori Algorithm. Apriori algorithm is mainly to mine some frequent item sets through generating the candidate sets and detecting the closed downward plots. It is generally composed of two steps: first, all possible frequent item sets are screened to meet the given minimum confidence, then the item sets with strong rules are remained.
- *K*-means. *K*-means algorithm is a clustering analysis algorithm based on some given distance, which respectively divides all datasets into many given clusters to meet each data belonging to the nearest cluster and the center of gravity without change. The specific flowchart of the algorithm is shown as Fig. 1.5.

For the semi-supervised learning, both unlabeled and labeled data are suitable for training where the unlabeled is suitable for large amounts while the labeled does for small amounts. It includes some extensions to the supervised learning, generally draws reasonable predictions through learning the internal structure of the data and predicts the labeled data through modeling unlabeled data. The common semi-supervised learning algorithms are as follows:

- Graph Inference. Given a graph in which some nodes are labeled, the graph inference algorithm infers the categories of those remaining unlabeled nodes through various priors of the given graph and their relations. The similarity between two nodes is drawn from the following three aspects: the consistency of node attributes, the consistency of local topological structures and the between-node path reachability, as shown in Fig. 1.6. Specifically, the local structures as well as node attributes are encoded as high-level features with graph convolution, while the between-node path reachability is abstracted as reachable probabilities of random walks [1].
- Laplacian Support Vector Machine. The Laplacian support vector machine algorithm is that the edge distribution geometric structure information of the labeled data and the unlabeled data is converted into the manifold regularization terms, which are added to the traditional support vector machine algorithm. For this algorithm, the introduction of manifold regularization terms is the highlight, and simultaneously its objective function is composed of three terms as follows.

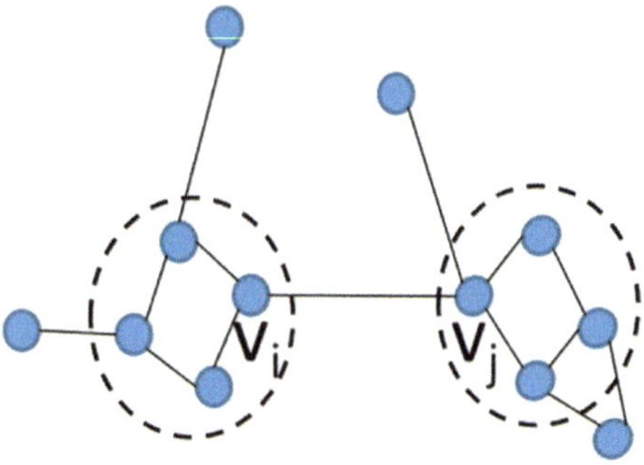

Fig. 1.6 Illustration of graph inference learning framework

$$\underbrace{f^*}_{\text{objective function}} = \arg\min_{f \in H_k} \underbrace{\frac{1}{l}\sum_{i=1}^{l} V(x_i, y_i, f)}_{\text{risk function}} + \underbrace{\gamma_A \| f \|_K^2}_{\text{regularization term}} + \underbrace{\gamma_I \sum_{i,j=1}^{l+u} \left(f(x_i) - f\left(x_j\right)\right)^2 W_{ij}}_{\text{manifold regularization term}} \tag{1.3}$$

The error and the trial search, along with the reward system, are the dominant characteristics of reinforced learning, which is a goal-oriented learning method through interaction, and uses the reward and punishment sequences to form an action strategy in a specific problem space. The common reinforced learning algorithms are as follows:

- Q-Learning. Q-Learning is a valued-based algorithm in the reinforced learning algorithm, i.e., $Q = Q(s, a)$ is defined as the expectation of the rewards, where $a \in A, s \in S$, A is an action set and S do a state set, then a Q-table is constructed to store the Q value, and finally the greatest reward is obtained through selecting the suitable action. The update process of Q-table is realized through the Eq. (1.4), where r is the reward, γ is the learning rate and α is the rewarding decay coefficient. Q-table of the Q-Learning algorithm is shown as Fig. 1.7.

$$Q(s, a) \leftarrow Q(s, a) + \alpha\left[r + \gamma \max_{a'} Q\left(s', a'\right) - Q(s, a)\right] \tag{1.4}$$

- State-Action-Reward-State-Action (SARSA). The decision-making procedure of the SARSA is similar as the above Q-Learning, where the unique difference lies in the following Eq. (1.5).

$$Q(s, a) \leftarrow Q(s, a) + \alpha\left[r + \gamma Q\left(s', a'\right) - Q(s, a)\right] \tag{1.5}$$

Q-Table	a1	a2
s1	q(s1,a1)	q(s1,a2)
s2	q(s2,a1)	q(s2,a2)
s3	q(s3,a1)	q(s3,a2)

Fig. 1.7 *Q*-table of *Q*-learning algorithm

1.2.3 Application of Machine Learning in Healthcare

In the recent years, the integration of machine learning and healthcare has arisen huge social influence in the prevention and treatment of diseases. Several typical examples of machine learning in healthcare are shown as follows.

Early warning of diseases. The early warning modeling of diseases based on machine learning can effectively improve the early diagnosis rate, reduce the warning time and enlarge the monitoring scope. It is also conductive for the medical institutions to take preventive and control measures, reduce disease deterioration and complications. First, index data or risk factors related to the disease are collected, then a model to discover the relationship between the pathogenesis and the disease hidden state is established. For examples, Tayefi et al. [2] established a predictive model for coronary heart disease using a decision tree algorithm, which need to enter 10 variables of a total 12 variables into the decision tree algorithm (including age, sex, fasting blood glucose, thyroglobulin, hypersensitive C-reactive protein, total cholesterol, high-density lipoprotein, low-density lipoprotein, systolic blood pressure and diastole pressure), and serum hypersensitive C-reactive protein levels is at the top of the tree, following by fasting blood glucose, gender and age. Their experiments have proved that the above model is accurate, specific and sensitive. Easton et al. [3] built a predictive classification models of post-stroke mortality, and found risk factors for the differences between short and longer term post-stroke mortality by naive Bayes of wide range variables across different time ranges, which is helpful for the patients' follow-up monitoring.

Chronic diseases research. Identifying risk factors of chronic disease such as diabetes, hypertension and cardiovascular disease and establishing warning models based on machine learning can help reduce the occurrence of chronic disease complications. For examples, Anjaiah et al. [4] implemented a heart disease prediction system using naive Bayes and K-means clustering algorithms, where K-means clustering algorithm was used to group various attributes (including age, gender, obesity, smoking, electrographic result, heart rate, chest pain, cholesterol, blood pressure and blood sugar) and identify risk factors for heart disease, then naive Bayes was utilized to diagnose whether the user is having heart disease or not and the preventive measures were taken. Tanvir Islam et al. [5] built up some rules using the Apriori algorithm with various diabetes symptoms and factors to predict diabetes efficiently.

Assisted medical diagnosis. Medical data are not only large in size, but also intricate and interrelated in content. The analysis of medical data and mining of valuable diagnostic rules based on machine learning will provide references for disease diagnosis. For example, Becerra-Garcia et al. [6] applied support vector machine algorithm to preprocess signals, detect impulses and mine data on electrooculograms, providing a basis for studying the identification of nonspontaneous saccades in clinical electrooculography tests. Yang et al. [7] proposed a method based on machine learning to analyze the correlation between the clinical information and pathology reports, and support the diagnosis of lung cancer pathological stage, so as to avoid surgical methods to obtain lung tissue during diagnosis. In this work, many attributes in the clinical data were obtained and classified by decision tree method, then the association rules among the attributes were extracted by Apriori algorithm, and the significance for medical diagnosis of each rule was examined using support, confidence and lift.

Disease gene prediction. Numerous studies have found that genes play a crucial role in the research of complex human diseases. Identifying the relationship between genes and diseases based on machine learning is important for improving the treatment of complex diseases. For examples, Nguyen et al. [8] presented a novel method to effectively predict disease genes by exploiting, in the semi-supervised learning scheme, data regarding both disease genes and disease gene neighbors via protein–protein interaction network. The findings were beneficial in deciphering the pathogenic mechanisms of chronic diseases. Cui et al. [9] utilized Q-learning algorithm of reinforced learning to propose the computational predictive model for human microRNA disease. The three submodels were used, collaborative matrix factorization (CMF), neighborhood regularized logistic matrix factorization (NRLMF), and Laplacian regularized least squares (LapRLS), which were fused via Q-learning algorithm to obtain the optimal weight S. The proposed model has better predictive performance of microRNAs by using eight diseases for local verification and carrying out case study on three common human diseases.

Telemedicine platform construction. Machine learning has made video detection in telemedicine platform very easy. With the help of machine learning, machine are programmed to observe the video cameras and detect any unusual behaviors. The machine will alert the person presenting in the surveillance cameras, which helps to remotely monitor people's abnormal behaviors. While the singular value decomposition algorithm can be used for medical images compression in remote transmission. For example, Forkan et al. [10] collected daily monitored vital signs data such as heart rate, average blood pressure, respiratory rate, blood oxygen saturation, and established disease warning models with decision tree algorithms. It is used for remote home monitoring to identify the occurrence of undiagnosed diseases, and send the monitoring results to medical emergency institutions to help the construction of telemedicine platform.

1.3 Deep Learning

1.3.1 Introduction

Deep learning is one of the broader machine learning based upon the neural networks, which lets the computer do what humans do through learning examples. The most apparent form of deep learning is the data passage through multiple layers, wherein the data become more abstract and more composite, so big labeled data and strong computing power are needed. In deep learning, the computer will take inputs or learn from sound, images, or text, perform the action with high accuracy accordingly, and implement it with computer vision, speech recognition, network filtering, social media, etc.

1.3.2 The Working Mechanism

There are numerous hidden layers in the neural network in deep learning. The common neural networks may contain around three hidden layers, where the deep and complicated networks may have more than 150 hidden layers. A large set of neural network architectures and labeled data allow the machine to learn the features. There are three common kinds of deep neural networks:

- Artificial Neural Networks (ANN).
- Convolution Neural Networks (CNN).
- Recurrent Neural Networks (RNN).

In most cases, deep learning is made feasible using ANNs that mimic neurons and brain cells. ANNs comprise three layers: input layer, hidden layer and out layer. Data is filled into the input layer, the hidden layer processes the input and the out layer generates the result. Figure 1.8 shows the basic structure of ANNs. Inputs are accorded with a specific weight and interlinked nodes enlarge the link's weight in the data process. The weight update uses the gradient descent method, that is, the weight is updated along the negative direction of the gradient to reduce the function value. The hidden layer is added with activation functions to avoid grid degradation. The output of each node is an activation of the weighted sum of inputs, which helps the network learn any complex nonlinear relationship between input and output. If the data unit reaches a specific threshold, it can pass on to the following layer. Figure 1.9 shows the specific learning process. To obtain information from experience, machines compare outputs from a neural network, then proceed to change connections, thresholds, and weights based on the variances among outputs.

CNNs are a very common kind of deep neural networks, which involves many learned features from input data and images through two-dimensional layers. The convolution kernel is an operator with learnable parameters, which is used to extract the features of the input image, and its output is usually a feature map. Figure 1.10

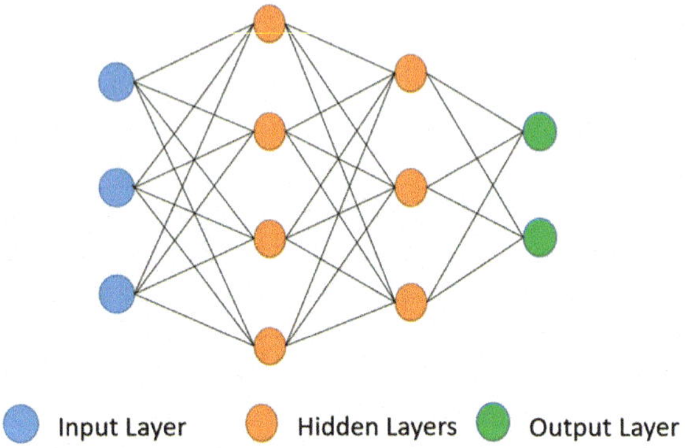

Fig. 1.8 Basic structure of artificial neural networks

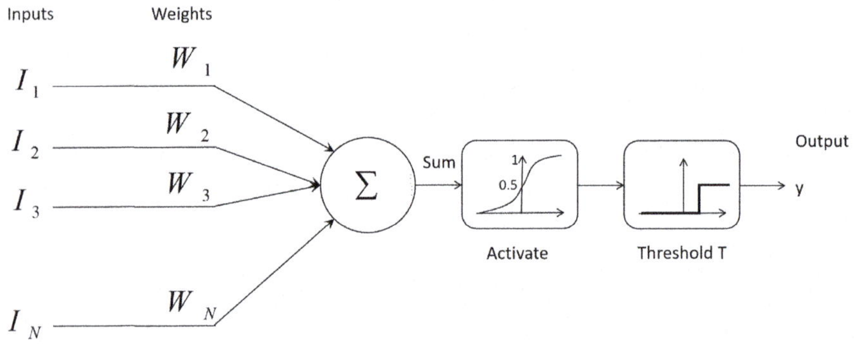

Fig. 1.9 Specific learning process of artificial neural networks

shows the specific process of feature map generation and output feature map size calculation equation can be expressed as (1.6). Therefore, there is no requirement for manual feature extraction and location in CNNs. In addition, CNNs may detect multiple features of an image with the multiple hidden layers, which will add much more complexity to the learned image features. For example, the first hidden layers can detect edges, the next ones will detect more complicated shapes until the whole object is detected. As the network will train the images, which provides a lot of accuracy in deep learning for object classification, some relevant features might not be needed.

$$F_0 = \left(\frac{F_{in} - k + 2p}{s} \right) + 1 \tag{1.6}$$

k: kernel size, p: padding size, s: stride

RNNs are neural networks structure for sequence data. Different from traditional ANNs, RNNs introduce directional loops, which can deal with the correlation

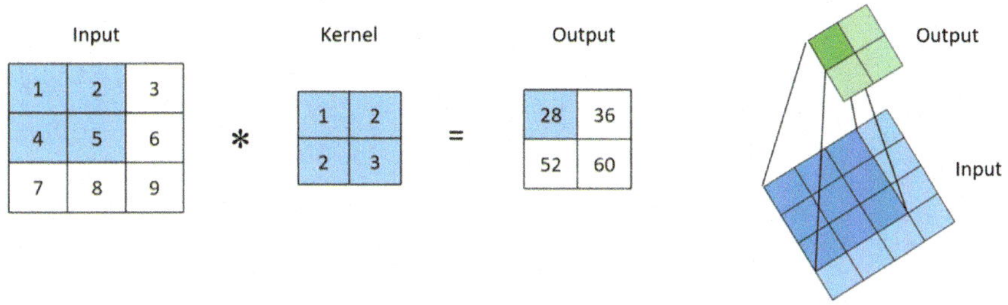

Fig. 1.10 Specific process of feature map generation

between inputs. Figure 1.11 shows the structure of RNNs, in which the current output of a sequence is related to the previous output. The core of RNNs is to cyclically use network layer parameters to avoid a sharp enlargement in parameters caused by increasing time steps. The specific expression is that the network will memorize the previous information and apply it to the calculation of the current output, that is, the nodes between the hidden layers are connected, and the input of the hidden layer not only includes the output of the input layer but also includes the output of the hidden layer at the previous moment. Figure 1.12 shows the calculation process of the network, where the three weight matrices U, W, V are weight matrices shared in all time steps, x_t represents the input of step t, s_t is the state of step t of the hidden layer with $s_t = f(Ux_t + Ws_{t-1})$, and o_t is the output of step t with $o_t = \text{softmax}(Vs_t)$.

Fig. 1.11 Structure of recurrent neural networks

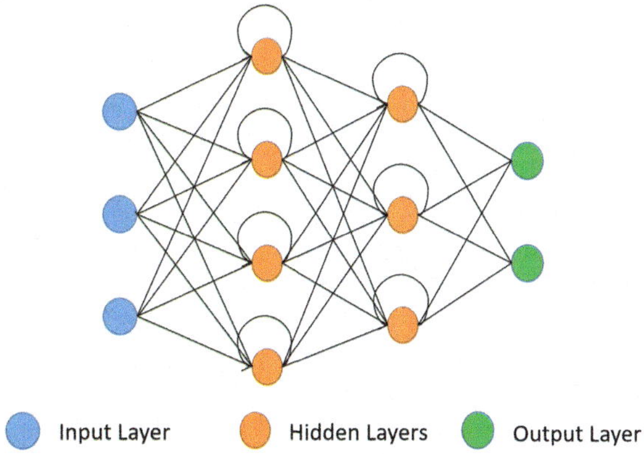

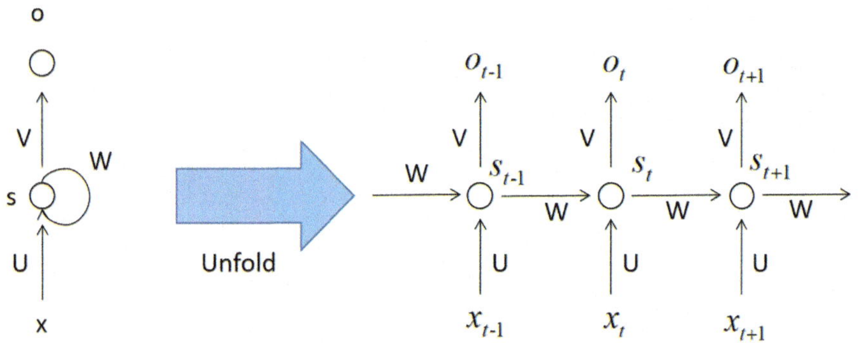

Fig. 1.12 Calculation process of recurrent neural networks

1.3.3 Deep Learning Models and MATLAB

There are three common ways to use deep learning to classify the object:

- Training from scratch.
- Transfer learning.
- Feature extraction.

For a network to be trained in deep learning, there is a need for many labeled data sets and the network architectural design that will be learning the model's features. This can be very effective and beneficial for the latest applications and applications that have multiple output categories. This approach is uncommon due to the longer training period, big data and leaning rate.

Transfer learning is a very common approach to deep learning, which has the ability to recognize and apply knowledge and skills learned in previous domains/tasks to novel domains/tasks. The ability is concretely to transfer high-quality labeled data or knowledge structure from related fields, and then complete or improve the learning effect of the target field or task. Figure 1.13 shows a classification method of transfer learning. Pre-training + fine-tuning is a very popular trick in deep learning, especially in the image filed. For example, pre-trained ImageNet is selected to initialize the model, which includes the fine-tuning. After a few changes in the network, the new task can be performed. This approach needs fewer data processing, therefore the computation time will be less than the previous approach. In addition, there is a need for an interface in transfer learning of the pre-existing network. There are good chances of modification and enhancement of the new task. The tools of MATLAB are specifically developed in transfer learning.

Feature extraction is not a very common approach for deep learning, which is only to use the feature extractor as all the layers are assigned to learn the special features from the images. These features can be pulled out from the network at any given time during the training process and can be used as a mode of input in the machine. A good example is the support vector machines.

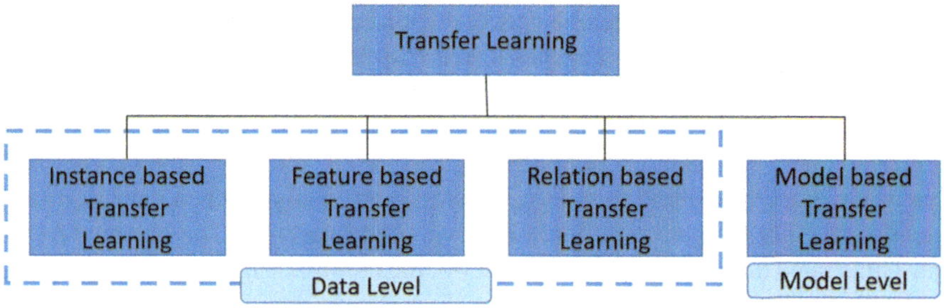

Fig. 1.13 Classification of transfer learning

Deep learning has been made very easy by MATLAB, which can help us in deep learning with a few code lines and offer a quick start by creating and visualizing the model and embedding the application model or the device. Using MATLAB has the characteristics as follows, i.e. there is no required expertise, their deep learning models have fewer codes and import the pertained models for debugging the initial results as the training parameters are adjusted.

Similarly, MATLAB can also be used to obtain expertise, learn about the special field and help domain experts in deep learning. For the images, it will enable the user to label the objects and combine different domains in one workflow. Moreover, it also gives different tools for deep learning and a long-ranged domains fed in deep learning algorithms, such as signal processing, data analysis, and computer vision. In addition, it also helps in integrating the outcomes in the existing applications and automates the deep learning models on embedded machines, clouds, and enterprise systems.

1.3.4 Application of Deep Learning in Healthcare

Deep learning is a method used to analyze and provide a learning process in big data analysis, which is constantly reshaping healthcare, medicine and life sciences, whether it is diagnosing skin cancer, bio-bank data or personalized medicine. Deep learning innovations are carving the future with precision medicine and health management in different ways. The following are a few examples of deep learning applications in healthcare that are currently getting known.

Analysis and prediction of diseases. The healthcare industries collect amounts of data that can contain some hidden information, which is useful for making effective decisions. The establishment of prediction systems of diseases based on deep learning can effectively predict the risk level of diseases and benefit early disease analysis, patient care and community services. For example, Singh et al. [11] developed an effective heart disease prediction system using neural network for the risk level of heart disease, which used 15 medical parameters such as age, sex, blood pressure, cholesterol, and obesity for prediction. Simultaneously, they employed the multi-layer perceptron neural network with back propagation as the training algorithm. The experimental results showed that the system predicts heart disease with 100% accuracy by using the neural network. Chen et al. [12] proposed a new multimodal disease risk prediction (CNN-MDRP) algorithm based on the convolution neural network using structure and unstructured data from hospitals. They used stochastic gradient method to train parameters, and finally reached the risk assessment of whether the patient suffered from cerebral infarction. The obtained results have illustrated that the prediction accuracy of the proposed algorithm reaches 94.8% with a faster convergence speed.

Detection of cancer cells. Discovering cancer at an early stage is an effective way to increase the chance of survival. However, since most screening processes are done manually, it is inefficient and thus a costly process. One way of automating the screening process could be to classify cells using deep learning techniques. CNNs in deep learning have been proven to be accurate for image classification tasks. Horie et al. [13] constructed the CNN system for detecting esophageal cancer. They used a deep neural network architecture called Single Shot MultiBox Detector which is a deep CNN that consisted of 16 layers or more and used a Caffe deep learning framework to train, validate, and test. When the trained CNN detected esophageal cancer from the input data of the test images, a disease diagnosis (superficial or advanced esophageal cancer) was assigned, and a rectangular frame was displayed in the endoscopic image so as to surround the lesion of interest. This system can detect stored endoscopic images in a short time with high sensitivity. In another case, invasive brain cancer cells cannot be visualized during surgery, so they are not removed. In vivo Raman spectroscopy can detect these invasive cancer cell in patients with grade 2 to 4 gliomas. But accurate detection was always becoming difficult due to spectral artifacts generated by lights in operating rooms. Jermyn et al. [14] have found that ANNs can overcome these spectral artifacts using nonparametric and adaptive models to detect complex nonlinear spectral characteristics. Coupling ANN with Raman spectroscopy simplifies the intraoperative use of Raman spectroscopy, detects the brain cancer cell more easily, and lowers the rate of residual cancer.

Construction of electronic health records. Electronic health records (EHRs) are rapidly becoming popular. Large medical institutions have collected EHR of more than 10 million patients in the past decade, which contain huge potential value. Therefore, applying deep learning methods to EHR data can quickly and efficiently tap the existed values. For an example, Khedkar et al. [15] discussed an attention mechanism and RNNs on EHR data for predicting heart failure of patients and providing insights into the key diagnoses. The patient's EHRs were given as a sequential input to the RNN which predicted the heart failure risk and provided his solutions. Here, a two-level neural network with attention mechanism model was designed to train the EHRs for detecting the patient's visits. When a prediction was drawn, the visit-level contribution was prioritized. The experiments showed that this proposed model can be effective for predicting the heart failure risks.

Robotic-assisted surgery. Robotic-assisted surgery using deep learning techniques promises to revolutionize surgery, including safer, more consistent and minimally invasive intervention. The important challenge of the robotic-assisted surgery is semantic segmentation of robotic instruments, which means correctly detecting an instrument's position for the tracking and pose estimation in the vicinity of surgical scenes. For an example, Shvets et al. [16] described the deep learning-based approach for robotic instrument segmentation, which was originally based on the combination of U-Net network architecture and the state-of-the-art semantic segmentation neural networks. The experiments demonstrated highly competitive performance for multi-class robotic instrument segmentation, and all networks can be used in an end-to-end pipeline, and performed efficient analysis on the full-resolution images.

Disease genome. Modern genome technology collects all kinds of measurement data, not merely from the DNA sequences of an individual to the content of various proteins in the blood. A genomic deep learning modeling has many opportunities to improve the methods used to analyze the above data, and ultimately helps clinicians provide more accurate treatments and diagnoses. Its typical analysis process mainly includes: obtaining raw data (such as gene expression data), converting the raw data into the data tensors, and then providing supports for specific biomedical applications. Recently, Sundaram et al. [17] trained a deep neural network by using thousands of common variants from population sequencing of six nonhuman primate species. The proposed network can identify pathogenic mutations in rare disease patients with 88% accuracy, and further advance the clinical utility of human genome sequencing.

1.4 Differences Between Machine Learning and Deep Learning

The comparisons between machine learning and deep learning are as follows:

- Data dependencies.
- Hardware dependencies.
- Problem-solving approach.
- Feature engineering.
- Execution time.
- Interpretability.

Table 1.1 shows the main differences between machine learning and deep learning.

1.4.1 Data Dependencies

Machine learning is the exploration of historical data called training data through computer programs. The major difference on deep learning for data dependencies is its performance as it increases with its scale, while it will not perform well when the data is in a small form. That is why deep learning requires a huge amount of data to deduce it perfectly. Dissimilarly, machine learning algorithms with their rules prevail in this case. Figure 1.14 shows this fact.

Table 1.1 Machine learning and deep learning differences

	Machine learning	Deep learning
Data dependencies	Excellent performances on a small or medium dataset	Excellent performances on a big dataset
Hardware dependencies	Low-end machines	High-end machines
Feature engineering	Need to understand the features that represent the data	No need to understand the best feature that represents the data
Execution time	From a few minutes to hours	Up to weeks
Interpretability	Easy to interpret	Difficult even impossible to interpret

Fig. 1.14 Differences in data dependencies

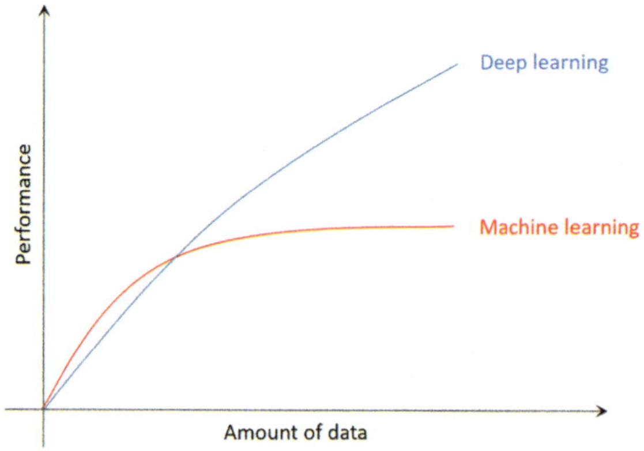

1.4.2 Hardware Dependencies

The deep learning algorithms need high-end machines, in contrast to machine learning algorithms, which can work on low types of machines. The reason behind the deep learning algorithm with high-end machines is that they include GPUs, an important part of how they work. When a large number of matrix multiplications are operated, GPUs can effectively optimize these operations.

1.4.3 Problem-Solving Approach

For the machine learning, we solve problems through breaking the problem into chunks so that every part can be solved separately, and then combine them to get the result. Although deep learning is a substrate of machine learning, it advocates solving problems from beginning to end on the contrary. As in the example below, when identifying which objects are on the image and find their locations, the machine learning will divide the problem into two steps: finding objects and recognizing objects. First, we have several box detection algorithms for object edges that frame all possible objects. Then, use object recognition algorithms, such as Support Vector Machine (SVM), to identify what these objects are. But deep learning is different that it directly identifies the corresponding object, and simultaneously indicates the name of the corresponding object for the given image.

1.4.4 Feature Engineering

Feature engineering is the process of creating domain knowledge into the feature extractors to reduce data complexity and make features more visible to learn. For machine learning, these features need to be identified by experts themselves and then hand-encoded according to the domain and data types. For example, features can be pixel value, shape, texture, position and orientation. The performance of most machine learning algorithms depends on what accurate feature identification and feature extraction are. As compared to machine learning, deep learning is an appropriate technique for separating important highlights from crude information and does not rely on hand-created highlights. In particular, it carries out a progressive element extraction, which learns highlights layer-wise, that is, it adapts to low-level highlights in beginning layers. As it climbs the chain of command, it becomes familiar with a progressively conceptual portrayal of the information.

1.4.5 Execution Time

Deep learning usually needs time to learn. This is because that there are many parameters where learning takes longer than usual. When a lot of data need to be dealt with, learning with essential data takes time. Additionally, when the number of layers in the designed network increases, the number of parameters known as the weight will increase, which will lead to slow learning. Not only the learning, but deep neural networks can take a long time to construct because testing will pass through all the layers. Machine learning normally costs a few hours even a longer time, depending on the applications and modeling outcome requirements. For example, the state-of-the-art deep learning ResNet takes about two weeks to train due to a massive data analysis, whereas machine learning comparatively takes much less time to train because of less analytical processes.

1.4.6 Interpretability

For the machine learning, the exact rules are given by the algorithm to explain the decision behind a specific option, so it is easy to interpret their expectations. But for a deep neural network, each layer represents a feature, and if there are more layers, what features they represent may not be known at all, and the trained model cannot be used to explain the prediction task. In addition, although the nerve cells which are active are understood, what a specific neuron is doing in the exact quantified manner, what these nerve cells need to do and what the nervous layer are cannot be known.

1.5 Artificial Intelligence in Healthcare

AI technology in the healthcare industry is undergoing development at a swift pace and is already being put to use in numerous applications ranging from helping arriving at a diagnosis to enhancing operational healthcare workflow effectiveness. A good number of these application objectives are to carry out the activities assumed by human beings at an improved pace with increased accuracy and more reliability, making them prospectively beneficial in resource-limited settings with constrained access to medical professionals and additional health professionals. In the following sections, top uses of AI in the healthcare sector will be introduced.

1.5.1 Medical Diagnostics

AI improves medical diagnostics and imaging that is constructed to enhance the reliability and speed of evaluation and has the potential to be specifically beneficial in settings where there is a deficiency of radiologists or trained doctors. Many successful cases using AI technology, especially deep learning, have already been reported in the field of medical imaging diagnosis. AI-based computer-aided diagnosis (CAD) shows equal or even better performance than doctors themselves. In conventional CAD development, the designer struggles to devise and create feature quantities that should be recognized in the image, such as the shape and density information of the cancerous area. The advantage of AI is that it can create more excellent features by itself through its learning process. That is, conventional CAD follows the development process, as shown in Fig. 1.15a, AI-CAD using deep learning does through the development process shown in Fig. 1.15b, saving much time and efforts [18].

The mass screening of fundus photographs can be used to diagnose not only ophthalmic diseases such as glaucoma but also diabetic retinopathy and hypertensive retinopathy, for both hypertension and arteriosclerosis degree determination. For example, Poplin et al. [19] collected fundus photographs together with other medical care data from about 300,000 patients and predicted heart disease

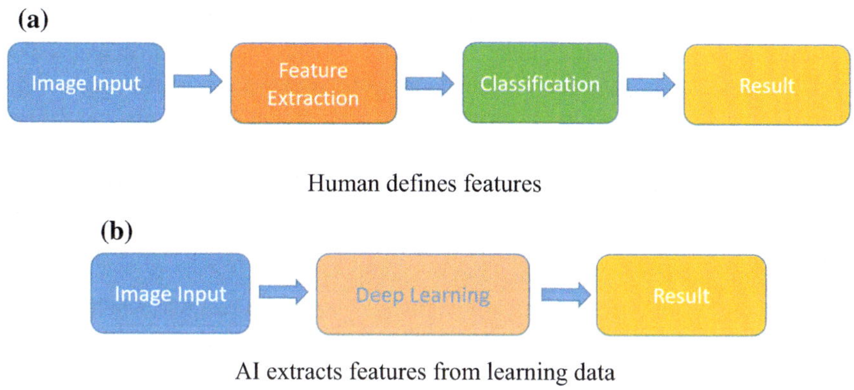

Fig. 1.15 **a** X Conventional CAD **b** Deep learning AI-CAD

using AI-CAD. They pre-processed the images for training and validation and trained the neural network. The optimization algorithm used to train the network weights was a distributed-stochastic-gradient-descent implementation. To speed up the training, batch normalization, as well as pre-initialization using weights from the same network trained to classify objects in the ImageNet dataset, was used. In addition, a technology called heat map was used to indicate the part of the fundus image that deep learning focuses on to make decision. Using deep learning processing, they predicted cardiovascular risk factors not previously thought to be present or quantifiable in retinal images, such as age, gender, smoking status, body mass index, systolic blood pressure, diastolic blood pressure and HbA1c. It can be said that this has already exceeded human work. A representative example of a single retinal fundus image for each prediction is shown in Fig. 1.16. We think that the attention mechanism can be introduced to further optimize the built deep learning network.

Risk Factors	Actual	Predicted
Age	57.6years	59.1years
Gender	female	female
Smoking	non-smoker	non-smoker
HbA1c	non-diabetic	6.7%
BMI	26.3 kg m^{-2}	24.1 kg m^{-2}
SBP	148.5mmHg	148.0mmHg
DBP	78.5mmHg	86.6mmHg

Fig. 1.16 Each prediction for a single retinal fundus image

AI for skin cancer diagnosis has also reached the same level as or higher than that accomplished by doctors. In January 2017, Esteva et al. [20] used AI to diagnose skin cancer. In their study, they demonstrated classification of skin lesions using a single CNN, and trained end-to-end from images directly, using only pixels and disease labels as inputs. They trained a CNN using a dataset of 129,450 clinical images and tested its performance with two critical binary classification use cases: keratinocyte carcinomas versus benign seborrheic keratoses, and malignant melanomas versus benign nevi. As a result, AI was able to diagnose skin cancer with accuracy equivalent to a dermatologist to some extent.

Even in the field of pathological imaging, AI's abilities can overwhelm against doctors. For an example, Bejnordi et al. [21] assessed the performance of automated deep learning algorithms at the detection and made a comparison of judgment results concerning the presence or absence of breast cancer lymph node metastasis for deep learning AI versus pathologists. By analyzing the presence of lymph node metastasis in an image, they rated their diagnostic as definitely normal, probably normal, equivocal, probably tumor, or definitely tumor. For the whole-slide image classification task, AI significantly performed better than the pathologists in a diagnostic simulation according to the comparison of the area under the receiver operating characteristic curve.

AI-based CAD system has also improved breast imaging classification and diagnostics, which is as accurate as experienced doctors. For an example, Wu et al. [22] presented a deep convolutional neural network for breast cancer screening exam classification, which was trained and evaluated on over 200,000 exams. They trained deep multi-view CNNs shown as Fig. 1.17, where the networks consisted of two core modules: four view-specific columns, each based on the ResNet architecture that output a fixed-dimension hidden representation for each mammography view, and two fully connected layers to map the computed hidden representations to the output predictions. The model concatenated L-CC (left craniocaudal) and R-CC (right craniocaudal) representations, and L-MLO (left mediolateral oblique) and R-MLO (right mediolateral oblique) representations. It made separate predictions for CC and MLO views, which were averaged during inference. Experiments showed that the proposed model was as accurate as experienced radiologists with the same data. In order to further improve the accuracy of the model, we consider replacing the ResNet architecture with the DenseNet architecture.

Additionally in the field of chest imaging, AI's abilities can as well as, or even outperform physicians. For an example, Hwang et al. [23] developed a deep learning-based algorithm that can classify normal and abnormal major thoracic diseases using nearly 90,000 chest radiographs (CRs) and evaluated them for external validation using over 1000 CRs. They adopted a deep convolutional neural network with dense blocks comprising 5 parallel classifiers, where four classifiers were designed for each disease, and the final classifier was designed for classification of CRs with abnormal results reflecting any of the target diseases. Then, two types of losses were designed to train the network: classification loss and localization loss. Both CRs with and without annotations were used in training, and finally, for each input CR, the proposed algorithm output continuous value between 0 and 1 as the image-level

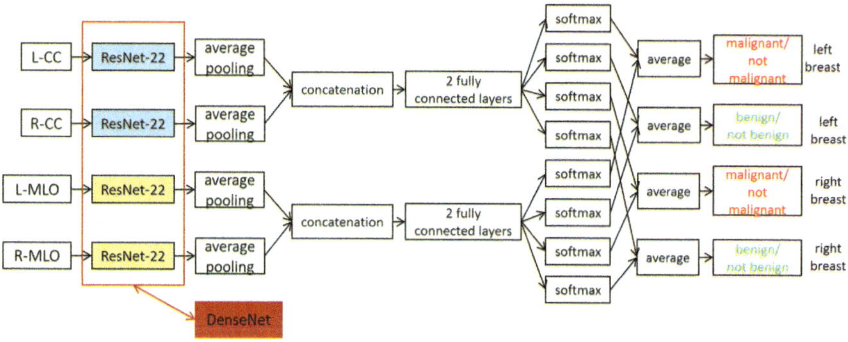

Fig. 1.17 Model for incorporating information across the four screening mammography views in an exam

probability of abnormal CR. The experiments showed that the algorithm consistently outperformed physicians in the discrimination of chest radiographs with major thoracic diseases and demonstrated its potential to improve the quality and efficiency of medical diagnostics.

AI autonomous diagnosis for COVID-19 has also achieved relatively remarkable results. Wang et al. [24] proposed multi-modal autonomous diagnosis algorithm of COVID-19 based on whale optimized support vector machine and improved D-S evidence fusion. Figure 1.18 shows the model of multi-modal autonomous diagnosis algorithm for COVID-19. The collected CT signals and experimental indexes are extracted to construct different feature vectors. The support vector machine is optimized by the improved whale algorithm for the preliminary diagnosis of COVID-19, and the basic probability distribution function of each evidence is calculated by the posterior probability modeling method. Then the similarity measure is introduced to optimize the basic probability distribution function. Finally, the multi-domain feature fusion prediction model is established by using the weighted D-S evidence theory. The experimental results show that the fusion of multi-domain feature information by whale optimized support vector machine and improved D-S evidence theory can effectively improve the accuracy and the precision of COVID-19 autonomous diagnosis.

1.5.2 Preconsulting Triage

AI triage pugs in telehealth settings and accordingly rea a pre-consulting triage, which further saves time by flagging prospective diagnosis for the physicians.

The use of AI appears to show significant promises in the emergency department triage in the present. The triage staging using AI can bring many benefits, such as accelerating diagnosis and optimizing workflow with few downsides. The ability to triage patients and take care of acute processes will largely benefit the health

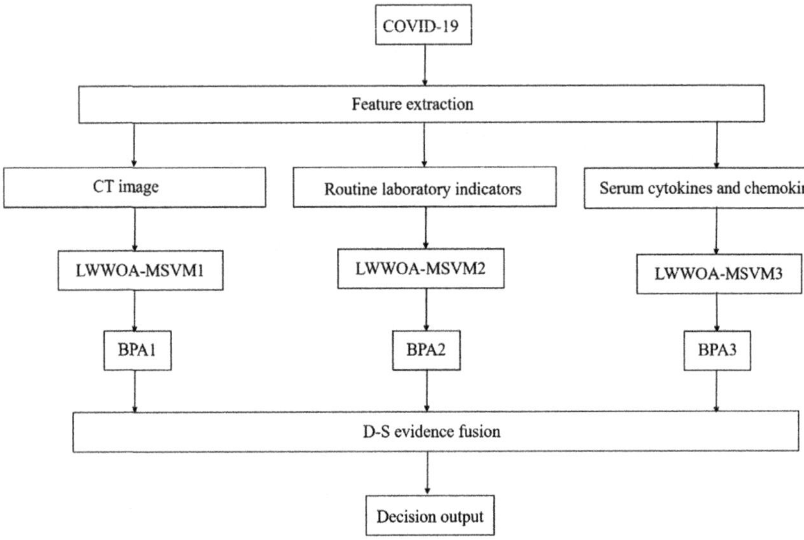

Fig. 1.18 Model of multi-modal autonomous diagnosis algorithm for COVID-19 [24]

system, improve patient care and reduce costs. For an example, Farahmand et al. [25] undertook the study to evaluate AI-based triage for patients with acute abdominal pain in the emergency department to estimate the emergency severity index version 4 (ESI-4) score, and developed a web-based interface (Fig. 1.19) using the models at the point of care. This interface firstly allowed quick entry of age, gender, vital signs and clinical signs, then the web interface passed these parameters to the prediction engine, and finally the prediction engine passed the input parameters to all models. Correspondingly, each model provided the ESI-4 score and the perceived accuracy of the result, and the prediction engine returned the result with the highest probability back to the web interface. The mixed-model approach using for predicting the ESI-4 score included association rules, clustering, logistic regression, decision trees, naive Bayes and neural networks. Before training the models, they used factor analysis to reduce the input variables. Seventy percent of the patient cases were used for training the models and the remaining 30% for testing the accuracy of the models. They compared the accuracy of the predictions between different algorithms and also compared with the emergency medicine physicians. The results showed that the application of AI in triage of patients with acute abdominal pains resulted in a model with the acceptable level of accuracy.

In the setting of the COVID-19 pandemic, AI may be used to carry out specific tasks such as pre-hospital triage and enable clinicians to deliver cares at scale. For an example, Lai et al. [26] implemented a digitally automated pre-hospital triage solution to allot patients to the appropriate care setting before they showed up at the emergency department and clinics, which would otherwise consume resources, expose

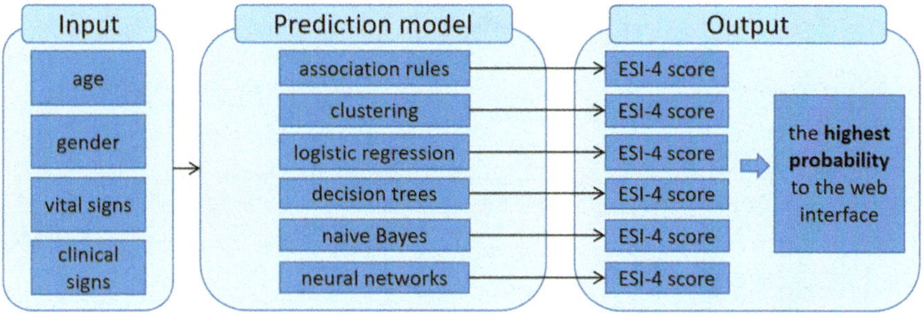

Fig. 1.19 Web interface for triage of the patients presented with acute abdominal pains

other patients and staff to potential virus transmission, and further exacerbate supply-and-demand mismatching. They developed a system of pre-hospital triage shown in Fig. 1.20, which would have to handle inquiries from existed patients, employees, and the general public through existed and new care settings. A standardized testing and triage algorithm would underlie the system to distinguish patients needing testing, patients safely reassuring to manage mild symptoms with self-quarantine at home and patients requiring more thorough medical evaluations and in-person cares. Therefore, they built a similar COVID-19 screener tool for patients seeking triage guidance, which uses a mobile-responsive, web-based interface to present users with a series of questions about risk factors and symptoms in order to capture the initial broad screening categories to determine whether the patient required additional consultation with a COVID-19 expert. The solutions fed a decision algorithm to arrive at a disposition endpoint. We think that the testing and triage algorithm used in the pre-hospital COVID-19 triage system could consider the mixed-model including clustering, logistic regression, decision trees, and naive Bayes.

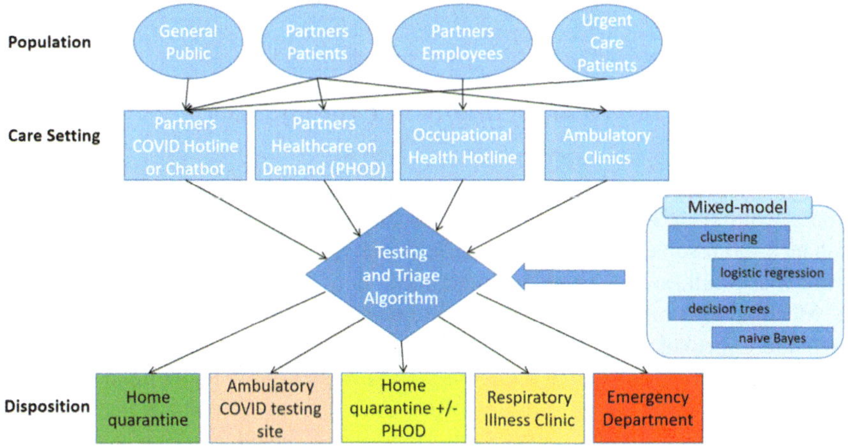

Fig. 1.20 Pre-hospital COVID-19 triage system

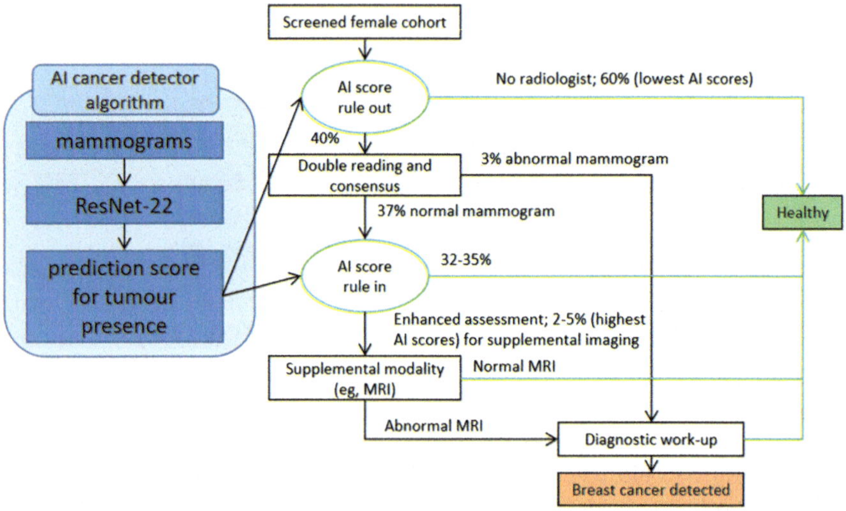

Fig. 1.21 Simulated triaging workflow

Even in the field of cancer detection, AI-based triage of cancer screening can promote early detection of cancers that would otherwise be diagnosed as interval cancers or next-round screen-detected cancers. For an example, Dembrower et al. [27] used the continuous prediction score between 0 and 1 of a commercial AI cancer detector algorithm to triage women into a no radiologist work stream when reaching to a score below a rule-out threshold, or into an enhanced assessment when doing a score above a rule-in threshold. They found that the above experiments could potentially reduce radiologist workload by more than half. Figure 1.21 describes the simulated AI triaging workflow. We consider replacing the deep neural network of the AI cancer detector algorithm with the ResNet in the future work.

1.5.3 Patient Information and Risk Evaluations

For machine learning and data analysis on the patient information such as electronic health data, AI gives promises to make it possible for predictive diagnosis and enhance the results in the long run. Additionally, AI looks at the human genome, which has 3 billion base pairs, and determines new medicines or health treatments.

Machine learning algorithms applied to data in the EHR can highlight the great potential to provide automated risk stratification for cardiovascular diseases. There is an example to predict future cardiovascular events in patients with the peripheral artery disease (PAD) using EHR data. Ross et al. [28] developed a novel predictive model using machine learning methods on electronic health record data to identify which PAD patients are most likely to develop major adverse cardiac and cerebrovascular events. They used penalized linear regression and random forest algorithms to build predictive models. All EHR data from every patient at an institution are included and let the algorithm identify the remained variables. They performed nested cross-validation, and chose the best-trained model based on the F-measure, and balanced model precision and recall. A total of 7686 patients were utilized in learning the predictive models with almost 1000 variables, and the best predictive model accurately determined which PAD patients would go on to develop major adverse cardiac and cerebrovascular events.

The prevalence of delirium is as high as 73% among surgical ICU patients. Studies show that one-third of delirium cases can benefit from multifactorial preventive measures and treatments which use machine learning models on EHR data. For an example, Davoudi et al. [29] used the preoperative EHR data for developing machine learning models to predict delirium. The predictive analysis workflow is outlined in Fig. 1.22. They compared the performance among seven machine learning models on delirium prediction. They first applied a data cleaning step to reduce errors by removing the outliers and used down-sampling and the synthetic minority oversampling technique (SMOTE) algorithm to remedy the imbalance in the datasets. They also used the random forests model to rank the features in the model based on their mean reduction in Gini impurity index. Among the evaluated models, random forests and the generalized additive model outperformed the other models in terms of the overall performance metrics for delirium prediction. Thus, using machine learning models could show the previously overlooked socioeconomic features and surgeon experience for delirium prediction and help healthcare staffs in identifying patients at higher risk of such complications.

With the completion of the 2023 International Human Genome Project, the emerging term "genomic medicine" has indicated a new type of medical treatment that provides patients with optimal treatment options based on the genome information using machine learning and deep learning techniques. For an example, when focusing on lung adenocarcinoma with clinical information, Hamamoto et al. [30] combined RNA-seq and miRNA expression data from The Cancer Genome Atlas (TCGA), performed a multi-omics analysis using an autoencoder, and then subclassified patients according to survival. The classifier was designed based on estimated labels derived from patient subtypes using support vector machine. They further identified survival-related subtypes of nonsmall cell lung cancer from six categories of TCGA multi-omics datasets (miRNA, mRNA, DNA methylation, somatic mutation, copy number variation, and reverse phase protein array), and successfully separated the poor and good prognosis groups of lung cancer patients. Through the above studies, they could accurately predict the prognosis of lung cancer patients and provide optimal treatments.

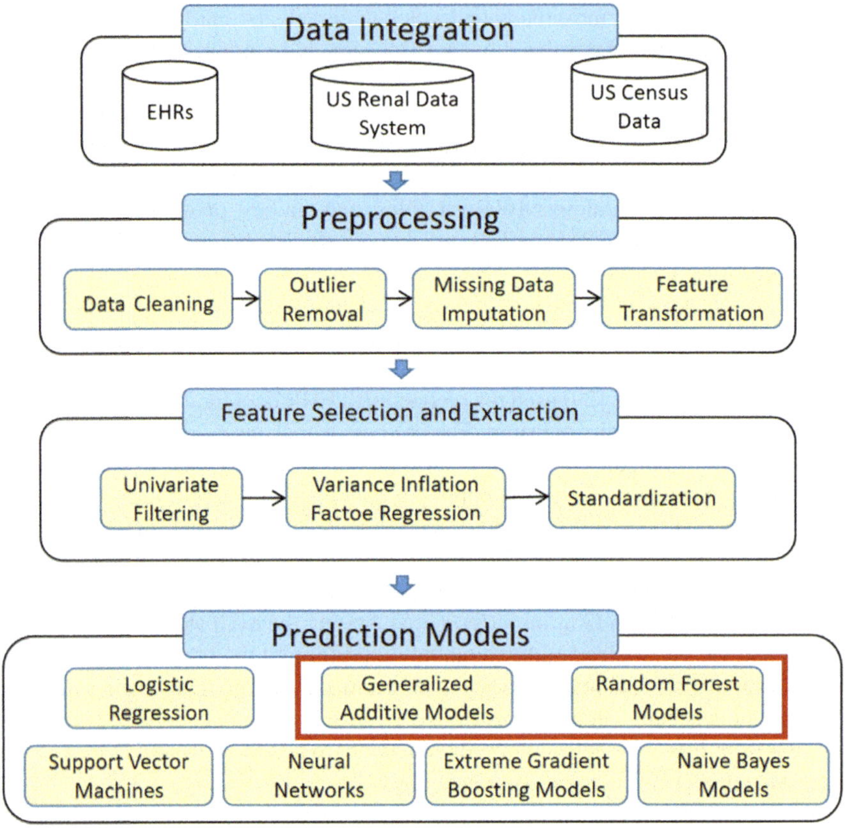

Fig. 1.22 Analysis workflow for prediction of delirium from EHR data

1.5.4 Discovery of Drugs

Deep learning methods that make use of convolutional neural networks happen to be very useful in predicting which molecular constructions end up yielding efficient drugs. AI likewise offers the support for personalized medicine and targeting medicines founded on personal genetics and additional genomic evaluation.

AtomNet [31] is a deep learning model that predicts the bioactivity of small molecules for drug discovery applications by using CNNs. It is known as the first major introduction of the deep learning technology into the prediction of protein–ligand interactions by using 3D protein structure information. Izhar Wallach et al. used network architecture of an input layer, followed by four 3D-convolutional layers and two fully connected layers with 1024 hidden units, each which were implemented with the ReLU activation function, and topped by a logistic-regression cost layer over two activity classes. AtomNet uses the complex structures of target proteins and small molecules, which are voxelized into a cube of 20 Å. To represent the structure of a protein–ligand complex, the environment of the atoms in the 3D structure is encoded into the fixed form of the feature vectors and the input layer receives vectorized versions of 1A 3D grids, which is showed in Fig. 1.23. By incorporating structural target information, AtomNet can predict new active molecules for targets.

Prediction of protein–ligand interactions is a critical step during the initial phase of drug discovery. Graph convolutional neural networks can serve as valuable tools in drug discovery. For an example, Son et al. [32] proposed the GraphBAR, a novel deep-learning-based prediction model based on a graph convolutional neural network, for protein–ligand binding affinity. Here, the structure of a protein–ligand complex is represented as a graph of multiple adjacency matrices whose entries are affected by distances, and a feature matrix that describes the atomic properties of the molecules. Figure 1.24 shows the scheme of graph representation with the structural database.

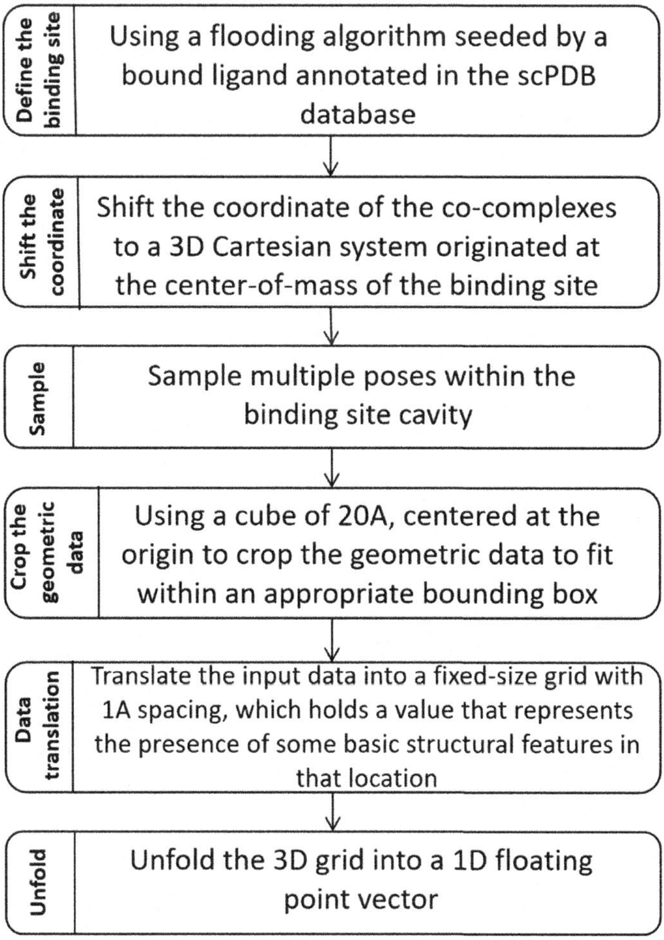

Fig. 1.23 Workflow of input representation in AtomNet

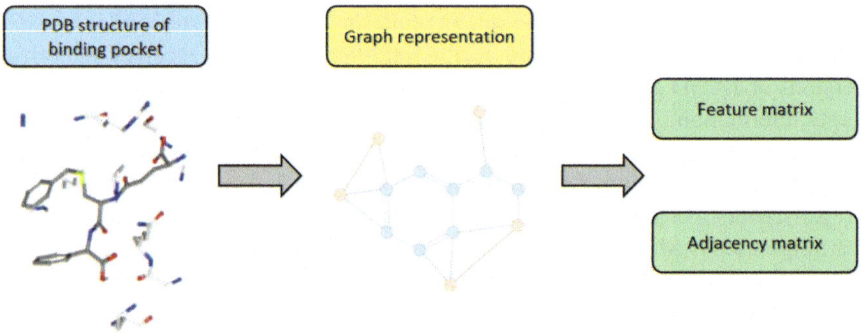

Fig. 1.24 Graph representation of protein–ligand binding structure

The architecture of the proposed model is illustrated in Fig. 1.25. The inputs of the model are one feature matrix and multiple adjacency matrices. First, the input feature matrix is processed by the fully connected layer and the dropout layer. Features extracted from these layers are fed into the different graph convolution blocks with one of the adjacency matrices. The graph convolution block has three graph convolution layers, composed of a fully connected layer and a dropout layer among them. The output of the last graph convolution layer is connected to the graph gather layer, which sums all the node feature values to create features representing the entire graph. All the outputs of the graph convolution blocks are concatenated, followed by the fully connected layer with the dropout layer and output layer for binding affinity prediction. GraphBAR has the high prediction performance for protein–ligand binding affinities by evaluation.

1.5.5 Pharmaceutical Supply Chain

The pharmaceutical supply chain [33] involves a complex network of steps required to produce a drug, from sourcing and supplying of materials, warehousing, manufacturing and distributing, to the drugs' end delivery to the pharmacy and patient. Figure 1.26 shows the main components of the pharmaceutical supply chain.

There's no shortage of AI solutions in the pharmaceutical market. Looking at the supply chain specifically, we're seeing a growing number of AI-led technologies offering solutions to many of the current challenges faced by the industry. Making use of AI to process real-time information and come up with predictive endorsements is supposed to drive data-motivated supply chains, thereby enhancing effectiveness and cost management.

For example, some programs can independently monitor market signals and accurately predict risks related to medicine shortages; others are using machine learning to control and reduce pharmaceutical costs and using real-time signals to direct when to buy and recommend formulary strategies [34]. As can be seen from the previous

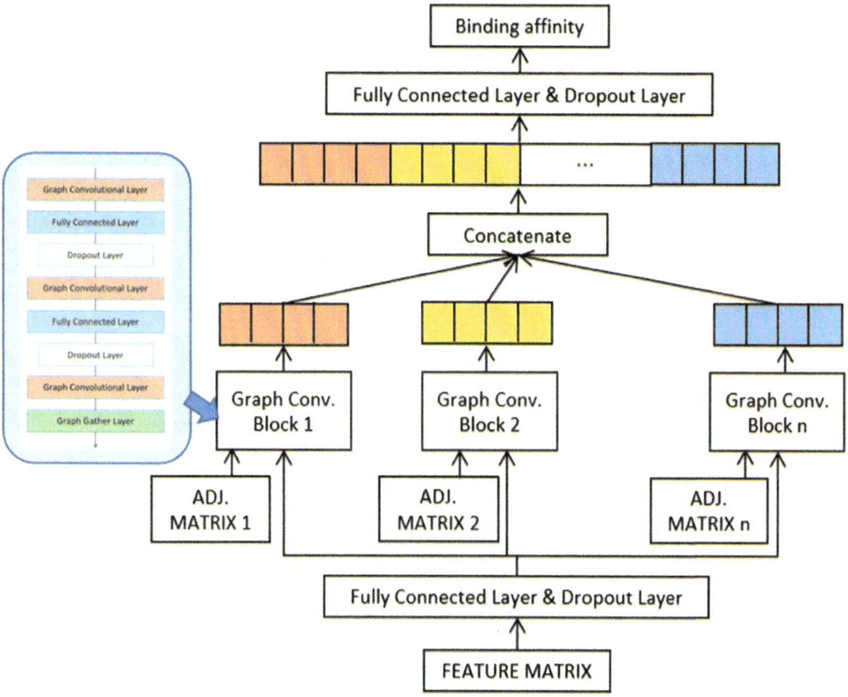

Fig. 1.25 Overview of the GraphBAR architecture

subsection, machine learning in bio-manufacturing for pharmaceuticals is ripe for optimization. Data from experimentation or manufacturing processes have the potential to help pharmaceutical manufacturers reduce the time needed to produce drugs, resulting in lowered costs and improved replication.

AI technologies can also being applied to predicting an imminent large-scale outbreak around the world, based on data collected from satellites, historical information on the web, real-time social media updates, and other sources, and giving local authorities and healthcare systems more time to react. The opioid epidemic is a direct live example of AI technology being utilized [35]. Support vector machines and artificial neural networks have been used to predict malaria outbreaks, with taking into account data such as temperature, average monthly rainfall, total number of positive cases, and other data points. Sudheer et al. [36] also proposed a novel method based on coupling the Firefly Algorithm (FFA) and SVM to forecast the malaria incidences. In this study, FFA has been employed for determining the parameters of SVM. The proposed SVM-FFA model has been adopted in predicting the malarial incidences in Jodhpur and Bikaner area where the malaria transmission is unstable, and provides more accurate forecasts compared to the other traditional techniques. Figure 1.27 shows a schematic clue depicting the SVM-FFA methodology. In the future work, we consider mix least squares support vector machine and

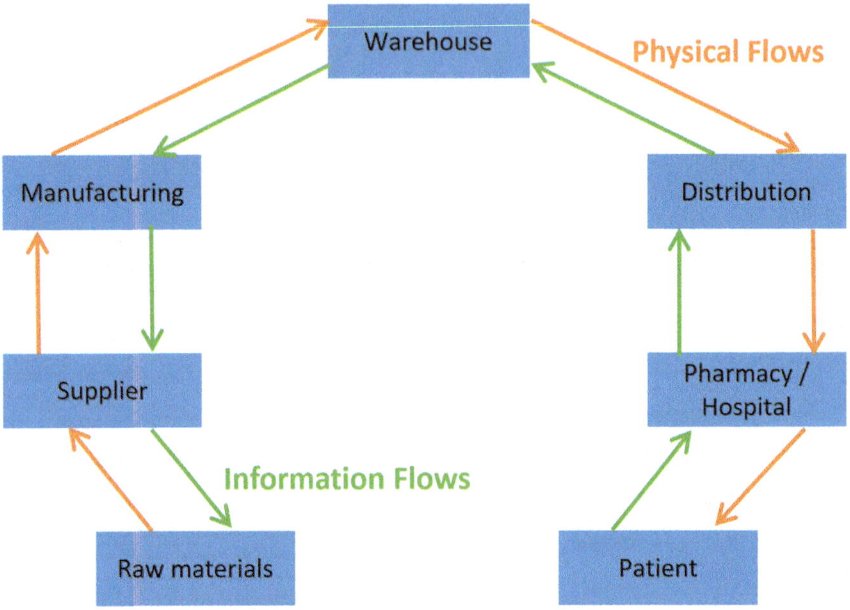

Fig. 1.26 Pharmaceutical supply chain

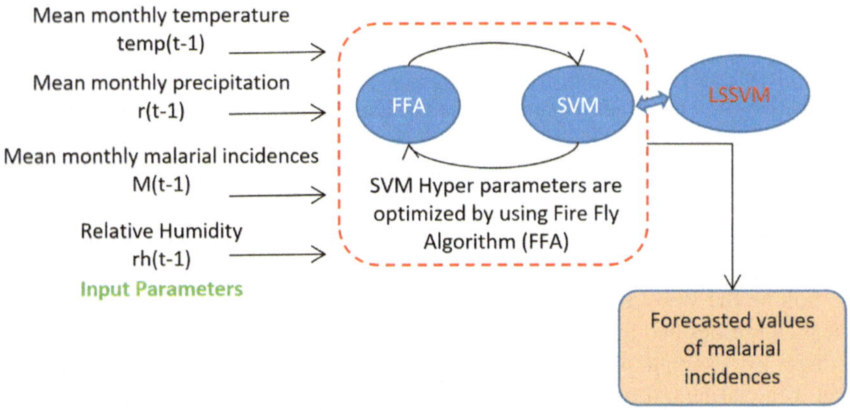

Fig. 1.27 Schematic picture depicting the SVM-FFA methodology

FFA to improve the accuracy of prediction. Furthermore, ProMED-mail [37] is an internet-based reporting program for monitoring emerging diseases and providing outbreak reports in real time. Leveraging ProMED reports and other mined media data, the organization HealthMap uses automated classification and visualization to help monitor and provides alerts for disease outbreaks in any country. Figure 1.28 shows the ProMED-mail information flowchart.

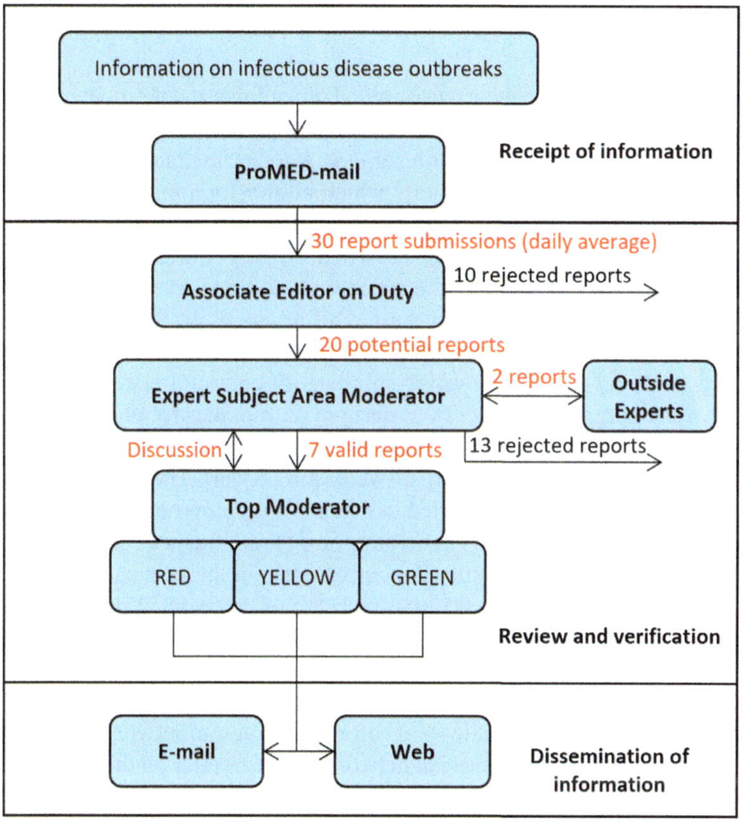

Fig. 1.28 ProMED-mail information flowchart

When it comes to transportation, AI is making it possible to predict and manage transportation capacity at a highly granular level, while virtually eliminating manual work and best-guess decisions.

A manufacturing line that focuses on quality brings even more advantages, such as reducing waste and minimizing risks, and can eliminate errors early in the drug development process. Combining AI with other advanced technologies can create a transparent, secure system and shield from counterfeit and substandard drugs. For an example, Ting et al. [38] constructed a deep learning drug identification model that distinguishes the authenticity of the drugs automatically using visual images of blister packages. They used the Faster R-CNN network, which is composed of two modules, where the first module which is a deep fully convolutional network proposes regions, and the second which is the Fast R-CNN detector uses the proposed regions.

1.5.6 Surgery Assistance

AI-assisted robotics can analyze past surgical procedures and their outcomes, which are allowed to guide surgeons on new or better practices, and have led to a 21% reduction in a patient's hospital stay after a surgery. Another use that is taking advantage of AI is image analysis in the surgery, which allows for a much quicker analysis. And AI can find things that humans just cannot discern.

AI can change practice in robot-assisted surgery toward cognitive surgical robotics, which will understand its environment and may even learn from experience to improve its performance over time. In research, AI-based robotic systems have been developed for situation-aware automatic needle insertion [39]. Riccardo Muradore et al. developed innovative solutions to control a novel robot designed to perform the surgical actions. They designed a modular robotic platform based on a macro/micro-unit architecture, consisting of two decoupled robotic structures that can be controlled independently as well as in concert. The proposed high-level control architecture, which is reported in Fig. 1.29, is composed of five components such as motion planner, trajectory generator, variable admittance control, robot driver and supervisor. In order to identify the current state in the surgical procedure from the real-time sensor data and a priori knowledge of the surgical plan, a three-layer supervised machine learning engine is implemented, with the upper-layer inferring with Bayesian networks, the middle-layer Gaussian clustering with a hidden Markov model and the lower-layer sensor filtering. Active filters are used to reduce the noise of the lower-layer to an acceptable level before the Bayesian networks and the hidden Markov model. The trained Bayesian network is able to infer on the real-time input, which is shown in Fig. 1.30a, while the real-time discrete input states such as the force state and the needle tip distance to the target are obtained by the hidden Markov model (HMM) layer which is shown in Fig. 1.30b. The experiments demonstrated that the proposed system was able to intervene the cryoablation of the kidney tumor, execute the needle insertion and monitor the procedure.

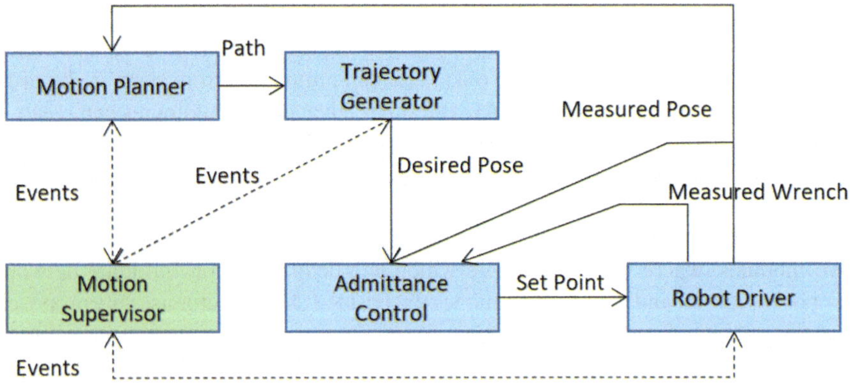

Fig. 1.29 Interconnection scheme of robot motion planning and control components

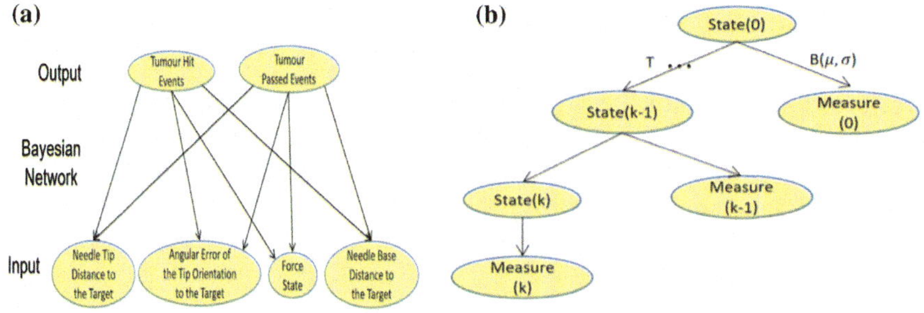

Fig. 1.30 **a** X Bayesian network **b** Sequence of observable states in the HMM

In surgery, machine learning-based algorithms are being studied for use as decision aids in risk prediction and even for intraoperative applications, including image recognition and video analysis. With modern deep learning designs, the analysis of live endoscopic images in surgery can be realized which is demonstrated in a recent article. Tokuyasu et al. [40] developed an intraoperative landmark indication system that outlined the landmarks on endoscopic images in real time using YOLOv3, which is an algorithm for object detection based on deep learning and predicts an objective score for each bounding box using logistic regression shown in Fig. 1.31. Using YOLOv3, the colored bounding boxes showed the respective position and class of each landmark, including cystic duct, common bile duct, lower edge of the left medial segment and Rouviere's sulcus. The use of intraoperative landmark indication systems will help reduce the incidence of bile duct injury, and increase the safety of laparoscopic cholecystectomy. In future work, we could consider introducing Gaussian model into YOLOv3 to improve accuracy.

Fig. 1.31 Bounding boxes with dimension priors and location prediction [40]

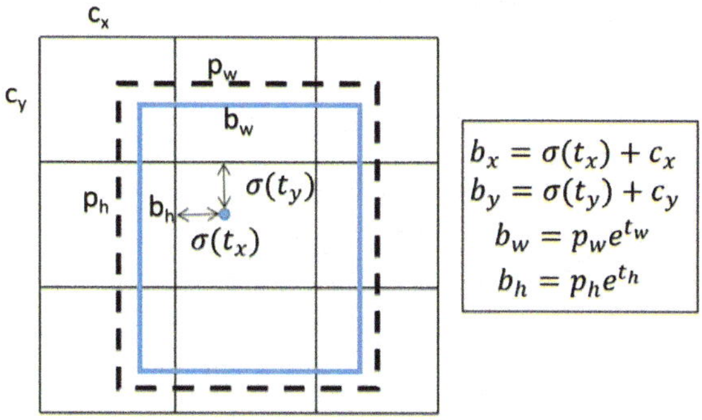

1.6 Challenges of Artificial Intelligence

The idea of AI is to take extremely lager amounts of data and make intuitive and fast decisions that will lead to greater efficiency and productivity. AI also does not have a perfect track record and still makes mistakes as it is just a machine. Sometimes a bug can be small and cause little problems, or large and do big issues. Even though the use of AI strategies in healthcare has great potential, it also brings especially daunting challenges in the healthcare sector. Some of the challenges need to be managed with wisdom as follows.

1.6.1 Data Quantity and Quality

The quality of any system is reliant on the kind of input data. AI systems in healthcare need enormous training datasets and more data than human beings in order to pinpoint patterns. The more improved the data given, the more enhanced the results will be provided.

1.6.2 Gathering Data

The data gathered by AI systems must come from reliable sources, otherwise come to bias and adversely affect the output of an AI solution. Healthcare organizations also need to prepare accurate datasets for machine learning algorithms, which is often difficult to overcome. They also need to ensure data is aligned with the building process and make their data compatible by cleaning the data to minimize missing values and eliminate irrelevant data.

1.6.3 Eliminating Black Box

As AI systems are "black box" models, an inevitable conclusion is arrived at like a prediction but lacks an explanation. Blindly trusting AI solutions can put patients' lives at risk. These systems can augment transparency by using explainable AI to help researchers understand the output and indicate the decision parts. One of the most common methods is the back propagation method, which is a widely used AI algorithm for supervised training of feedforward neural networks. The implementation of this explainable AI approach will ensure patient and physician trust in AI conclusions.

1.6.4 Model Accuracy

If an AI system makes a mistake, it becomes hard to pinpoint the precise place. The above challenges can make AI generate outcomes and predictions that are deficient in precision and accuracy. In response to such challenges, experts have to come up with developments like Whitebox Testing, which is developed for deep learning systems. It is responsible for testing the neural network using a large number of inputs and pinpoints, at which point the reactions are faulty and need to be mended.

1.6.5 Evaluating Vendors

Healthcare organizations need multiple machines for diagnosis, which requires them to understand the complexities of different machines. So they need to wisely evaluate and choose AI vendors. It is a good idea to choose the most promising vendor in the form of a workshop. In this way, it will be possible to consult vendors on how to easily and quickly integrate AI solutions with specific machines, and then the right vendor will help healthcare organizations build AI solutions that integrate existing equipment and workflows.

1.6.6 Legal Matters

Medical staff at a hospital apply the AI system to provide needed care services for a patient. Then, should the responsibility of the AI be on the system design firm, hospital, or medical staff? This is a very difficult question to answer as it involves a number of technical, managerial and ethical issues. Dr. Stephen Hawking suggested that a new global governance agency must be established to regulate the use of AI [41]. Privacy issues arise in terms of data collection and sharing, which raises ethical, moral and legal issues. Healthcare organizations need to ensure that the collected data is protected to enhance privacy and security. The fusion of AI and blockchain can ensure secure transmission and storage of patient data and also provide transparency to patients so they can see where their data are stored and how they are being used.

1.6.7 Educating Staff and Patients

There are many benefits to leverage AI solutions, but using them is complex. Insufficient awareness of the AI potential and how to be harnessed can lead to skills gaps in organizations. Healthcare organizations need to bridge the skills gap by educating employees. Hospitals and experts can organize special training sessions in different departments to train employees on how to use AI systems. Healthcare organizations should raise awareness about the benefits of robotic surgery and can also educate patients about AI robotic surgical procedures before operating them. Educating patients and staff about AI solutions will ensure increased trust in AI systems.

References

1. Xu C, Cui Z, Hong X, Zhang T, Yang J, Liu W. Graph inference learning for semi-supervised classification [C]. International conference on learning representations (ICLR), 2020.
2. Tayefi M, Tajfard M, Saffar S, Hanachi P, Amirabadizadeh AR, Esmaeily H, Taghipour A, Ferns GA, Moohebati M, Ghayour-Mobarhan M. Hs-CRP is strongly associated with coronary heart disease (CHD): a data mining approach using decision tree algorithm[J]. Comput Methods Programs Biomed. 2017;141:105–9.
3. Easton JF, Stephens CR, Angelova M. Risk factors and prediction of very short term versus short/intermediate term post-stroke mortality: a data mining approach[J]. Comput. Biol. Med. 2014;54(C):199–10.
4. Anjaiah A, Reddy KR, Reddy RAK, Harshavardhan. Heart disease prediction system using k-means clustering and naïve bayes algorithm[J]. Int. J. Curr. Adv. Res. 2019;8(3):18001–03.
5. Tanvir Islam M, Raihan M, Farzana F, Ghosh P, Ahmed Shaj S. An empirical study on diabetes mellitus prediction using Apriori algorithm[C]. International conference on innovative computing and communications, 2020. p. 539–50.
6. Becerra-García RA, García-Bermúdez RV, Joya-Caparrós G, Fernández-Higuera A, Velázquez-Rodríguez C, Velázquez-Mariño M, Cuevas-Beltrán FR, García-Lagos F, Rodráguez-Labrada R. Data mining process for identification of non-spontaneous saccadic movements in clinical electrooculography[J]. Neurocomputing. 2017;250:28–36.
7. Yang H, Chen YP. Data mining in lung cancer pathologic staging diagnosis: correlation between clinical and pathology information[J]. Expert Syst Appl. 2015;42(15–16):6168–76.
8. Nguyen TP, Ho TB. Detecting disease genes based on semi-supervised learning and protein-protein interaction networks[J]. Artif Intell Med. 2012;54(1):63–71.
9. Cui L, Lu Y, Sun J, Fu Q, Xu X, Wu H, Chen J. RFLMDA: a novel reinforcement learning-based computational model for human microRNA-disease association prediction[J]. Biomolecules. 2021;11(12):1835.
10. Forkan ARM, Khalil I, Atiquzzaman M. ViSiBiD: a learning model for early discovery and real-time prediction of severe clinical events using vital signs as big data[J]. Comput Netw. 2017;113:244–57.
11. Singh P, Singh S, Pandi-Jain GS. Effective heart disease prediction system using data mining techniques[J]. Int J Nanomed. 2018;13:121–4.
12. Chen M, Hao Y, Hwang K, Wang L, Wang L. Disease prediction by machine learning over big data from healthcare communities[J]. IEEE Access. 2017;5:8869–79.
13. Horie Y, Yoshio T, Aoyama K, Yoshimizu S, Horiuchi Y, Ishiyama A, Hirasawa T, Tsuchida T, Ozawa T, Ishihara S, Kumagai Y, Fujishiro M, Maetani I, Fujisaki J, Tada T. Diagnostic outcomes of esophageal cancer by artificial intelligence using convolutional neural networks[J]. Gastrointest Endosc. 2019;89(1):25–32.
14. Jermyn M, Desroches J, Mercier J, Tremblay MA, St-Arnaud K, Guiot MC, Petrecca K, Leblond F. Neural networks improve brain cancer detection with Raman spectroscopy in the presence of operating room light artifacts[J]. J Biomed Opt. 2016;21(9):94002.
15. Khedkar S, Gandhi P, Shinde G, Subramanian V. Deep learning and explainable AI in healthcare using EHR[M]. Deep learning techniques for biomedical and health informatics. 2020. p. 129–48.

16. Shvets AA, Rakhlin A, Kalinin AA, Iglovikov VI. Automatic instrument segmentation in robot-assisted surgery using deep learning[C]. 2018 17th IEEE international conference on machine learning and applications (ICMLA). 2018. p. 624–28.
17. Sundaram L, Gao H, Padigepati SR, McRae JF, Li Y, Kosmicki JA, Fritzilas N, Hakenberg J, Dutta A, Shon J, Xu J, Batzoglou S, Li X, Farh KK. Predicting the clinical impact of human mutation with deep neural networks[J]. Nat Genet. 2018;50(8):1161–70.
18. Fujita H. AI-based computer-aided diagnosis (AI-CAD): the latest review to read first[J]. Radiol Phys Technol. 2020;13(1):6–19.
19. Poplin R, Varadarajan AV, Blumer K, Liu Y, McConnell MV, Corrado GS, Peng L, Webster DR. Prediction of cardiovascular risk factors from retinal fundus photographs via deep learning[J]. Nat Biomed Eng. 2018;2(3):158–64.
20. Esteva A, Kuprel B, Novoa RA, Ko J, Swetter SM, Blau HM, Thrun S. Dermatologist-level classification of skin cancer with deep neural networks[J]. Nature. 2017;542(7639):115–8.
21. Bejnordi BE, Veta M, van Diest PJ, van Ginneken B, Karssemeijer N, Litjens G, van der Laak JAWM, the CAMELYON16 Consortium, Hermsen M, Manson QF, Balkenhol M, Geessink O, Stathonikos N, van Dijk MC, Bult P, Beca F, Beck AH, Wang D, Khosla A, Gargeya R, Irshad H, Zhong A, Dou Q, Li Q, Chen H, Lin HJ, Heng PA, Haß C, Bruni E, Wong Q, Halici U, Öner MÜ, Cetin-Atalay R, Berseth M, Khvatkov V, Vylegzhanin A, Kraus O, Shaban M, Rajpoot N, Awan R, Sirinukunwattana K, Qaiser T, Tsang YW, Tellez D, Annuscheit J, Hufnagl P, Valkonen M, Kartasalo K, Latonen L, Ruusuvuori P, Liimatainen K, Albarqouni S, Mungal B, George A, Demirci S, Navab N, Watanabe S, Seno S, Takenaka Y, Matsuda H, Phoulady HA, Kovalev V, Kalinovsky A, Liauchuk V, Bueno G, Fernandez-Carrobles MM, Serrano I, Deniz O, Racoceanu D, Venâncio R. Diagnostic assessment of deep learning algorithms for detection of lymph node metastases in women with breast cancer[J]. J. Am. Med. Assoc. 2017;318(22):2199–10.
22. Wu N, Phang J, Park J, Shen Y, Huang Z, Zorin M, Jastrzebski S, Fevry T, Katsnelson J, Kim E, Wolfson S, Parikh U, Gaddam S, Lin LLY, Ho K, Weinstein JD, Reig B, Gao Y, Toth H, Pysarenko K, Lewin A, Lee J, Airola K, Mema E, Chung S, Hwang E, Samreen N, Kim SG, Heacock L, Moy L, Cho K, Geras KJ. Deep neural networks improve radiologists performance in breast cancer screening[J]. IEEE Trans Med Imaging. 2020;39(4):1184–94.
23. Hwang EJ, Park S, Jin KN, Kim JI, Choi SY, Lee JH, Goo JM, Aum J, Yim JJ, Cohen JG, Ferretti GR, Park CM, DLAD development and evaluation group. Development and validation of a deep learning-based automated detection algorithm for major thoracic diseases on chest radiographs[J]. J. Am. Med. Assoc. Netw. Open 2019;2(3):e191095.
24. Wang G, Guo S, Han L, Song X, Zhao Y. Research on multi-modal autonomous diagnosis algorithm of COVID-19 based on whale optimized support vector machine and improved D-S evidence fusion[J]. Comput Biol Med. 2022;150: 106181.
25. Farahmand S, Shabestari O, Pakrah M, Hossein-Nejad H, Arbab M, Bagheri-Hariri S. Artificial intelligence-based triage for patients with acute abdominal pain in emergency department; a diagnostic accuracy study[J]. Adv J Emerg Med. 2017;1(1): e5.
26. Lai L, Wittbold KA, Dadabhoy FZ, Sato R, Landman AB, Schwamm LH, He S, Patel R, Wei N, Zuccotti G, Lennes IT, Medina D, Sequist TD, Bomba G, Keschner YG, Zhang HM. Digital triage: novel strategies for population health management in response to the COVID-19 pandemic[J]. Healthc (Amst). 2020;8(4): 100493.
27. Dembrower K, Wåhlin E, Liu Y, Salim M, Smith K, Lindholm P, Eklund M, Strand F. Effect of artificial intelligence-based triaging of breast cancer screening mammograms on cancer detection and radiologist workload: a retrospective simulation study[J]. Lancet Digit Health. 2020;2(9):e468–74.
28. Ross EG, Jung K, Dudley JT, Li L, Leeper NJ, Shah NH. Predicting future cardiovascular events in patients with peripheral artery disease using electronic health record data[J]. Circ.: Cardiovasc. Qual. Outcomes. 2019;12(3):e004741.
29. Davoudi A, Ebadi A, Rashidi P, Ozrazgat-Baslanti T, Bihorac A, Bursian AC. Delirium prediction using machine learning models on preoperative electronic health records data[J]. Proc IEEE Int Symp Bioinf Bioeng. 2017;2017:568–73.

30. Hamamoto R, Suvarna K, Yamada M, Kobayashi K, Shinkai N, Miyake M, Takahashi M, Jinnai S, Shimoyama R, Sakai A, Takasawa K, Bolatkan A, Shozu K, Dozen A, Machino H, Takahashi S, Asada K, Komatsu M, Sese J, Kaneko S. Application of artificial intelligence technology in oncology: Towards the establishment of precision medicine[J]. Cancers(Basel). 2020;12(12):3532.
31. Wallach I, Dzamba M, Heifets A. AtomNet: a deep convolutional neural network for bioactivity prediction in structure-based drug discovery[J]. Comput. Sci. 2015.
32. Son J, Kim D. Development of a graph convolutional neural network model for efficient prediction of protein-ligand binding affinities[J]. Public Libr Sci One. 2021;16(4): e0249404.
33. Owczarek D. Inefficiencies in pharmaceutical supply chain cost. Leveraging AI in drug supply chain management [J/OL]. [2021–03–30]. https://nexocode.com/blog/posts/ai-in-drug-supply-chain/.
34. Scceu. Leveraging AI in the pharmaceutical supply chain [N/OL]. [2020 Jan 13]. https://scceu.org/leveraging-ai-in-the-pharmaceutical-supply-chain/.
35. Faggella D. 7 applications of machine learning in pharma and medicine [J/OL]. [2020 March 04]. https://emerj.com/ai-sector-overviews/machine-learning-in-pharma-medicine/.
36. Sudheer C, Sohani SK, Kumar D, Malik A, Chahar BR, Nema AK, Panigrahi BK, Dhiman RC. A support vector machine-firefly algorithm based forecasting model to determine malaria transmission[J]. Neurocomputing 2014;129:279–88.
37. Madoff LC. ProMED-mail: an early warning system for emerging diseases[J]. Clin Infect Dis. 2004;39(2):227–32.
38. Ting HW, Chung SL, Chen CF, Chiu HY, Hsieh YW. A drug identification model developed using deep learning technologies: experience of a medical center in Taiwan[J]. BMC Health Serv Res. 2020;20(1):312.
39. Muradore R, Fiorini P, Akgun G, Barkana DE, Bonfe M, Boriero F, Caprara A, Rossi GD, Dodi R, Elle OJ, Ferraguti F, Gasperotti L, Gassert R, Mathiassen K, Handini D, Lambercy O, Li L, Kruusmaa M, Manurung AO, Meruzzi G, Nguyen HQP, Preda N, Riolfo G, Ristolainen A, Sanna A, Secchi C, Torsello M, Yantac AE. Development of a cognitive robotic system for simple surgical tasks[J]. Int. J. Adv. Robot. Syst. 2015;12(4).
40. Tokuyasu T, Iwashita Y, Matsunobu Y, Kamiyama T, Ishikake M, Sakaguchi S, Ebe K, Tada K, Endo Y, Etoh T, Nakashima M, Inomata M. Development of an artificial intelligence system using deep learning to indicate anatomical landmarks during laparoscopic cholecystectomy[J]. Surg Endosc. 2021;35(4):1651–8.
41. Lee D, Yoon SN. Application of artificial intelligence-based technologies in the healthcare industry: opportunities and challenges[J]. Int J Environ Res Public Health. 2021;18(1):271.

Chapter 2
Artificial Intelligence and Blockchain

2.1 Introduction

Blockchain and AI are two of the most smoking innovation inclines at present. Even though the two advances have unique features in creating gatherings and applications, scientists have been talking about and investigating their mix, which have been found to go amazingly well together.

First, we should try to comprehend the idea of blockchain. A blockchain is a decentralized, open computerized record and is cryptographically secure. It is done using hashes that continually refer the chain's next block. This means that data can be shared but remains secure because if a hash is tampered with, it will not match all the following blocks. Creating new blocks with the rules allows for good security and data integrity.

Blockchain has three characteristics: immutability, decentralization and transparency. Decentralized units can handle higher measurements, resulting in very high-performance AI systems. Blockchain offers an open, shared and decentralized information databases that can be accessed and refreshed by those with authorization. Blockchain databases hold their data in an encoded state. This aspect implies that only private keys, a couple of kilobytes information, need remain secret for the majority information on the chain to be secure.

Information sharing is the principal advantage of blockchain for AI. When combining blockchain with AI, a reinforcement framework for the individual information is proposed. Putting away medicinal information on a blockchain, which can be reached by an AI using just authorization once it has experienced the correct techniques, could give us the gigantic favorable circumstances of customized proposals while securely putting away our touchy information.

As AI is related to information, blockchain turns into an entryway that prompts secure information exchange over the web. Blockchain ensures security among gadget correspondence. It also guarantees the information confirmation on which AI models depend on. Most forecasts and examples using AI and blockchain are

S. Guo et al., *Advanced Technologies in Healthcare*,
https://doi.org/10.1007/978-981-99-9585-1_2

increasingly exact compared to the information mining that AI performs, which generally utilizes fragmented, missing information. Also, among blockchain and AI, the error-prone human components are dispensed with.

Regardless of how AI offers enormous points of interest in numerous fields, if it is not trusted by the general population, at that point, its handiness will be severely constrained. With blockchain programming, all means from information passage to conclusions can be watched, which will ensure that this information has not been altered. This builds trust in the conclusions drawn by AI programs.

2.2 Core Technologies of Blockchain

The blockchain originated from bitcoin. During the formation of bitcoin, blocks are storage units one by one, which record all the communication information of each block node within a certain period of time. Each block is linked through random hashing (also known as hash algorithm), and the next block contains the hash value of the previous block. The result is called a blockchain. The linked list is composed of blocks in series, as shown in Fig. 2.1. To add new data, it must be placed in a new block. Whether this block (and the transactions in the block) is legal can be quickly checked by calculating the hash value. Any maintenance node can propose a new legal block, but must go through a certain consensus mechanism to reach a consensus on the final selected block.

The blockchain in the narrow sense is a chain data structure that combines data blocks in a sequential manner according to time sequence and is an untamperable and unforgeable distributed ledger guaranteed by cryptography. The generalized blockchain technology is a new distributed infrastructure that uses the blockchain data structure to verify and store data, uses distributed node consensus algorithm to generate and update data, uses cryptography to ensure the security of data transmission and access and uses smart contracts composed of automated script code to program and manipulate data.

Generally speaking, the blockchain system consists of data layer, network layer, consensus layer, incentive layer, contract layer and application layer. As shown in Fig. 2.2, the data layer encapsulates the underlying data blocks, related basic data and basic algorithms such as data encryption and time stamps; the network layer includes distributed networking mechanisms, data dissemination mechanisms and data verification mechanisms; the consensus layer mainly encapsulates various consensus

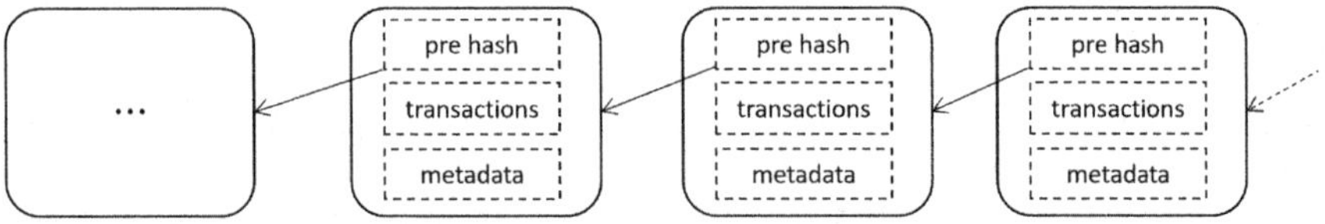

Fig. 2.1 An example of a blockchain structure

Fig. 2.2 Blockchain infrastructure model

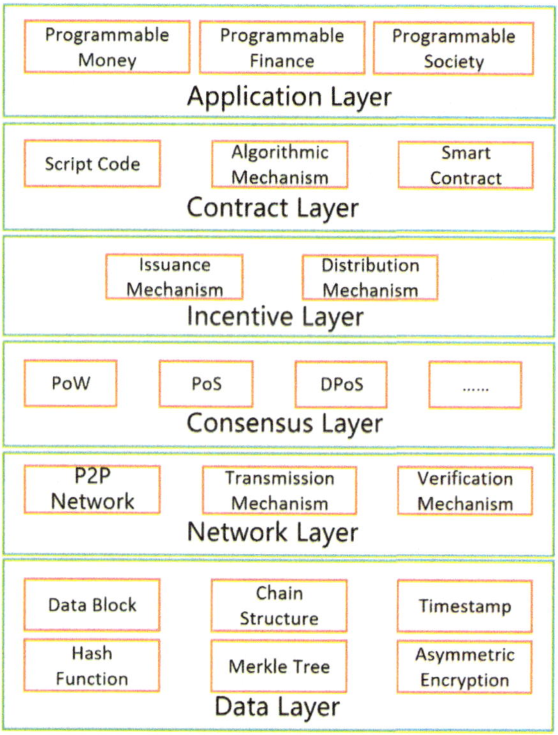

algorithms of network nodes; the incentive layer integrates economic factors into the blockchain technology system, mainly including the issuance mechanism and distribution mechanism of economic incentives; the contract layer mainly encapsulates various scripts, corresponding algorithms and smart contracts, which is the basis of the programmable features of the blockchain; the application layer encapsulates various application scenarios and cases of the blockchain. In this model, hash algorithm, consensus algorithm, asymmetric encryption algorithm, smart contract, distributed storage technology and P2P network technology are the core technologies of blockchain, which are described in details.

2.2.1 Hash Algorithm

The hash algorithm is constructed on the basis of the hash function, which can achieve fast forward, difficult reverse, input sensitivity and collision avoidance. The hash function can compress a message of any length into a fixed-length binary string within a limited and reasonable time, and its output value is called a hash value, which defines as $h = H(m)$, m is a message of any length, H is a hash function, and h is a fixed-length hash value.

$$Ch(x,y,z) = (x \wedge y) \oplus (\overline{x} \wedge z) \qquad Ma(x,y,z) = (x \wedge y) \oplus (x \wedge z) \oplus (y \wedge z)$$

$$\Sigma_0(x) = S^2(x) \oplus S^{13}(x) \oplus S^{22}(x) \qquad \Sigma_1(x) = S^6(x) \oplus S^{11}(x) \oplus S^{25}(x)$$

$$\sigma_0(x) = S^7(x) \oplus S^{18}(x) \oplus R^3(x) \qquad \sigma_1(x) = S^{17}(x) \oplus S^{19}(x) \oplus R^{10}(x)$$

Fig. 2.3 Logical functions in SHA256

SHA256 is a typical hash function that produces a 256-bit message digest for messages smaller than 264 bits, which first complete message padding and expansion padding, convert all input original messages into n 512-bit message blocks, and then use SHA256 compression function to process each message block. Its specific calculation steps are as follows:

Step 1: Constant initialization. 8 hash initial values ($h_0 - h_7$) and 64 hash constants are used in the SHA256 algorithm. The initial hash value is the first 32 bits in the fractional part of the square root of the first 8 prime numbers in the natural numbers, and then the hash constant is obtained by taking the first 32 bits in the fractional part of the cube root of the first 64 prime numbers in the natural numbers.

Step 2: Additional padding bits and additional length value. Padding at the end, it first fills the first bit with 1, and then fills with 0 until the length satisfies the remainder after modulo 512 is 448. Then it copies the length information of the original data (the message before padding) to the end of the message that has been padding.

Step 3: Logical operations. The operations involved in the SHA256 hash function are all logical bit operations, including the logical functions as shown in Fig. 2.3.

Step 4: Computational information digests. First, the message is decomposed into 512-bit blocks. Assuming that the message M can be decomposed into n blocks, all the algorithm needs to do is to complete n iterations. The result of n iterations is the final hash value, which is a 256-bit digital digest. The initial value H_0 of a 256-bit digest is calculated after the first data block to obtain H_1, that is, the first iteration is completed, and the processing is performed in sequence, and finally H_n is obtained, which is the final 256-bit message digest. In the first iteration, the initial value of the mapping is set to 8 initial hash values. The specific algorithm for each iteration is described below:

- Construct 64 words. For each block, the block is decomposed into 16 32-bit words, denoted as $w[0], \ldots, w[15]$, and the remaining words are obtained by the following iterative formula (2.1)

$$W_t = \sigma_1(W_{t-2}) + W_{t-7} + \sigma_0(W_{t-15}) + W_{t-16} \tag{2.1}$$

- Perform 64 cycles. One iteration is completed by performing 64 encryption cycles, and each encryption loop can be described by the Fig. 2.4, where the 8 words

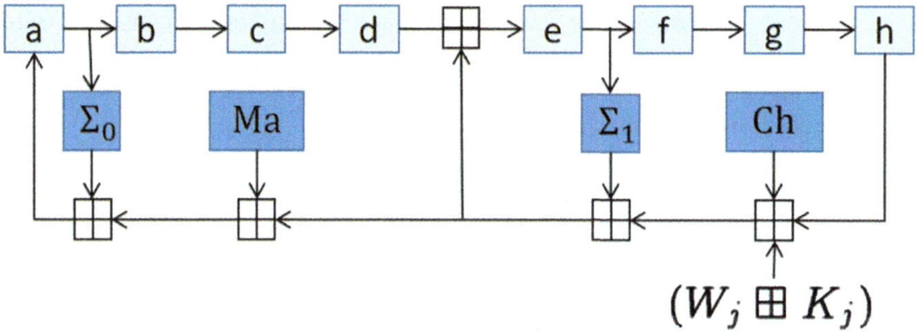

Fig. 2.4 Encryption loop in SHA256

ABCDEFGH are updated according to certain rules. The square represents adding two numbers together. If the result is greater than 2^32, it must be divided by 2^32 to find the remainder. K_t is the t-th key, corresponding to the 64 constants mentioned above, and W_t is the t-th word generated in this block.

Under the existing computing resources, it is not feasible to find two different messages with the same value under the same hash function. Hash functions have no convenient way to generate a hash value that satisfies special requirements, and their difficulty-friendliness forms the basis of proof-of-work-based consensus algorithms. The hash value that meets specific requirements can be used as proof of work in the consensus algorithm.

2.2.2 *Consensus Algorithm*

As a distributed system, blockchain is a network cluster composed of multiple host nodes through asynchronous communication. State replication is required between the nodes to ensure that the hosts reach a consistent state consensus. Therefore, the blockchain must solve the problem of consensus among nodes in distributed scenarios, and the consensus algorithm can be used to ensure the consistency and correctness of the data of different nodes in the system to different degrees. According to different blockchain types, consensus algorithms can be mainly divided into two categories. A type of consensus algorithm used in public chain scenarios, mainly including Proof of Work (PoW) algorithm, Proof of Stake (PoS) algorithm and Delegate Proof of Stake (DPoS) algorithm. For example, bitcoin adopts the method of solving the Hash256 mathematical problem, that is, the PoW algorithm, to ensure that the ledger data forms a correct and consistent consensus in the entire network. The other type is the consensus algorithm used in the consortium chain scenario, mainly including Byzantine fault-tolerant algorithms RBFT and RAFT. Different scenarios have different requirements for the efficiency and security of the consensus algorithm. It is the best choice to choose a suitable consensus algorithm and improve the consensus algorithm for suitable scenarios. Table 2.1 shows the main characteristics of these consensus algorithms.

2.2.3 Asymmetric Encryption Algorithm

The asymmetric encryption algorithm mainly uses the public key and the private key to encrypt and decrypt data storage and transmission. Its application scenarios in blockchain mainly include information encryption, digital signature and login authentication. The asymmetric encryption algorithms involved in the blockchain system mainly include RSA, D-H, and ECC (elliptic curve encryption algorithm). In the blockchain system, a pair of public key and private key is generated based on the asymmetric encryption algorithm. The public key is used to encrypt data, and the corresponding private key is used to decrypt data. On the contrary, the data encrypted with the private key is digitally signed, and decrypted with the corresponding public key is the signature verification. Taking the process of bitcoin transaction as an example, the public key is converted into an address for accepting bitcoin through a hash function, and the private key is used for transaction signature during bitcoin payment, which confirm that the payer will be the ownership of the bitcoin being traded at that moment.

Taking RSA algorithm as an example, RSA algorithm is the most widely used asymmetric encryption algorithm today. The encryption process of RSA can be expressed by a general Eq. (2.2)

$$\text{ciphertext} = \text{plaintext}^{E}\text{modN} \tag{2.2}$$

It can be seen from the above equation that anyone who knows E and N can perform RSA encryption, so E and N are the keys of RSA encryption, that is to say, the combination of E and N is the public key, we use (E, N) to represent the public key. The decryption of RSA can also be expressed by a general Eq. (2.3)

$$\text{plaintext} = \text{ciphertext}^{D}\text{modN} \tag{2.3}$$

where knowing D and N can decrypt the ciphertext, so the combination of D and N is the private key. Since the public key is (E, N) and the private key is (D, N), the key pair is (E, D, N), but how is the key pair generated? The steps are shown in Table 2.2.

Table 2.1 Consensus algorithm characteristics

	PoW	PoS	DPoS	RBFT	RAFT
Principle	The difficulty of generating a block is proportional to the computing power level of the current node in the network, and the entire network adopts the same mining difficulty	The difficulty of generating blocks should be proportional to the stake that the current node occupies in the network, and the difficulty of mining or generating blocks depends on the number of stakes	Shareholders grant voting rights to representatives, and the representatives with the most votes have equal internal powers and take turns to generate blocks	A message-passing-based consensus algorithm that achieves consensus through three phases may be repeated due to failure	All members elect a leader, and the leader is responsible for generating blocks
Feature	Nodes with large computing power may control the accounting rights in a short period of time	The gap between the rich and the poor is widening, and the richest man may dominate accounting rights	The improvement of PoS and the distribution of accounting rights in the rich club, no longer depend on computing power	When the number of failed nodes is less than m (total nodes are 3m + 1), the possible damage caused by the failed client can be limited	Strong leadership. Evil leaders are destructive, and leaders have a single point of performance bottleneck
Usage scenario	Node and computing power balance deployment Suitable for public chains	Participant negotiation Suitable for public chains	Permanent representative Not suitable for public chains	There are strong consistency requirements It is suitable for alliance chain and private chain	The leader is authoritative and suitable for private chains
Decentralization	Completely decentralized, nodes come in and out freely	Fully centralized	Close to centralization	Semi-centralized	Approximate centralization
Performance	Low	Low	High	High	High

Table 2.2 Generate key pair

N	$N = p * q$; p and q are prime number
L	$L = \mathrm{l\,cm}(p-1, q-1)$; L is the least common multiple of $p-1$ and $q-1$
E	$1 < E < L$, $\gcd(E, L) = 1$; The greatest common divisor of E and L is 1 (E and L are relatively prime)
D	$1 < D < L$, $E * \mathrm{DmodL} = 1$

2.2.4 *Smart Contract*

Smart contracts are divided into broad smart contracts and narrow smart contracts. A smart contract in a broad sense refers to a computer program running on the blockchain. A smart contract in a narrow sense runs on the blockchain infrastructure, based on agreed rules which is event-driven and has a state, and can save assets on the ledger. It is an automatically executable computer program using program code to encapsulate and verify complex transaction behaviors to achieve information exchange, value transfer and asset management. All mentioned in this book are narrow smart contracts. The common types of smart contracts include scripted smart contracts, turing-complete smart contracts, and verifiable contract smart contracts.

Taking the Ethereum development platform as an example, the smart contract operation mechanism mainly includes the following stages (shown in Fig. 2.5):

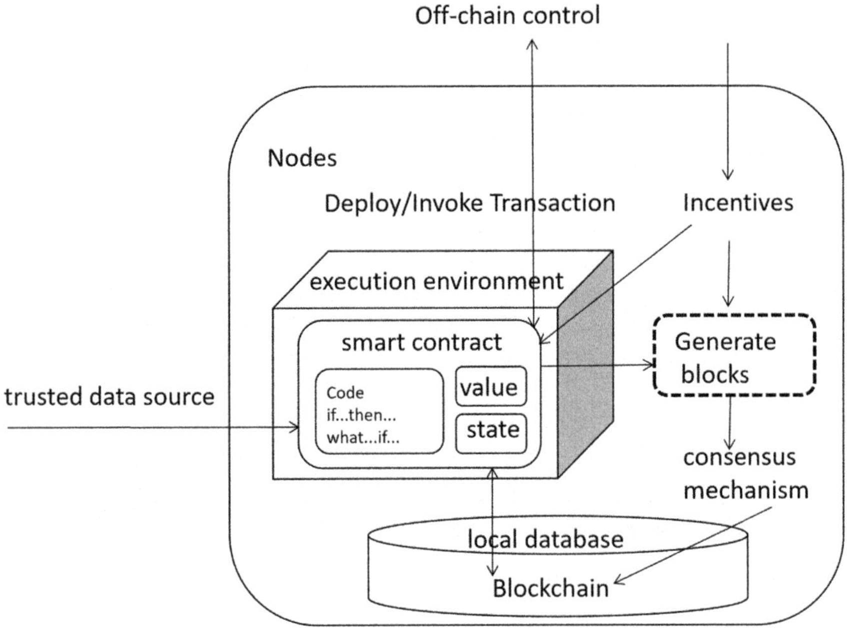

Fig. 2.5 Smart contract operation mechanism

- Code generation. Smart contracts generally have two attributes: value and state. The code uses If–Then and What–If statements to preset the corresponding trigger scenarios and response rules of the contract terms. On the basis that all aspects of the contract are agreed, the evaluation determines whether the contract can be implemented by a smart contract, i.e. "programmable", and then the content of the contract described in natural language will be translated into executable machine language by a programmer using a suitable development language.
- Compilation. Smart contract codes written in development languages generally cannot be run directly on the blockchain, but need to be executed in a specific environment. Therefore, before uploading the contract file to the blockchain, it is necessary to use the compiler to compile the original code to generate bytecode that meets the requirements of the environment.
- Submission. The submission and invocation of smart contracts are completed through "transactions". After the user initiates the submission of contract documents in the form of transactions, it broadcasts the entire network through the P2P network, and each node stores it in the block after verification.
- Confirmation. The verified valid transaction is packaged into a new block, and after reaching an agreement through the consensus mechanism, the new block is added to the main chain of the blockchain. The account address of the smart contract is generated according to the transaction, and then the account address can be used to invoke the contract by initiating a transaction. The node processes the verified and valid transaction, and the invoked contract is executed in the environment.

2.2.5 Distributed Storage Technology

Distributed storage-related technologies originate from the technologies in the process of data decentralized storage, including distributed storage, distributed computing, CAP theory, and consistency algorithms. This technology is used to solve the problems of data storage, backup, fault tolerance and consistency of distributed systems. As a distributed storage system, blockchain uses distributed storage technology. Based on distributed storage technology, the blockchain stores data in multiple independent nodes, and each node participates in the accounting and storage of the blockchain. Therefore, the risk of server crash that may occur in the data centralized storage mode is avoided. The high fault tolerance of the blockchain ensures that all built-in services of the system can be maintained stably and continuously from the beginning of operation, which greatly ensures the reliability and availability of the blockchain system.

Here, Inter Planetary File System (IPFS) is taken as an example to introduce the distributed storage architecture. IPFS is fully decentralized, and its working principle is shown in Fig. 2.6. The file, as well as all of the blocks within it, is given a unique fingerprint called a cryptographic hash. IPFS removes duplications across the network, and each of network node stores only content which it is interested in,

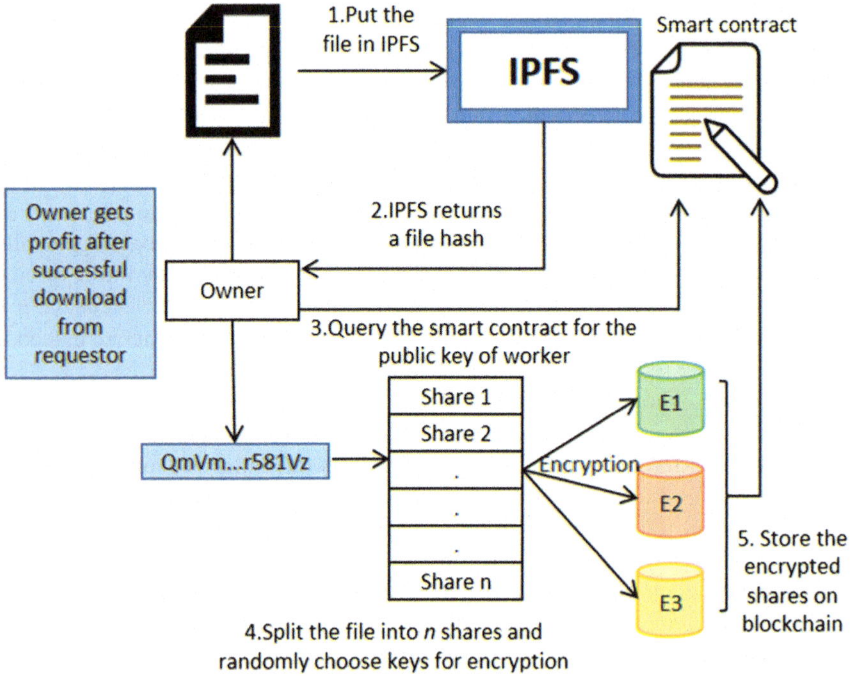

Fig. 2.6 Workflow of IPFS

plus some indexing information that helps figure out what the node is storing. When looking up a file to view or download, the network is asked to find the modes that are storing the content behind that file's hash. There is no need to remember the hash, though every file can be found by human-readable names using a decentralized naming system called IPNS.

2.2.6 P2P Network Technology

P2P is short for peer-to-peer, so P2P network technology is also called peer-to-peer network technology. P2P network technology is a networking technology that connects peer nodes in a blockchain system. As a distributed network, each node on the network can directly access each other without going through an intermediate entity, and simultaneously share its own resources, including storage capacity, network connection capacity, processing capacity, etc. Before the emergence of blockchain technology, P2P network technology has been widely used in many fields such as network video, network voice, search, and download. The communication and interaction of each node in the application of blockchain technology uses the

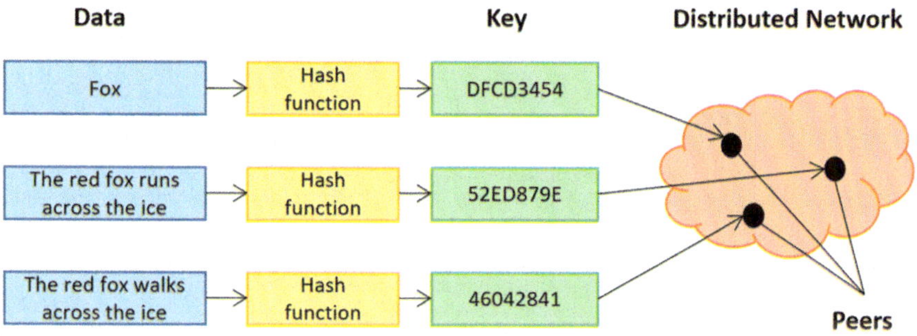

Fig. 2.7 Distributed hash table

relatively mature P2P network technology. Therefore, P2P network technology is one of the core technologies of blockchain.

P2P network is mainly divided into centralized network, fully distributed unstructured network, fully distributed structured network and hybrid network. At present, the most widely used is the structured distributed network, that is, the network based on DHT (distributed hash table). In order to achieve the efficiency and correctness of Napster and the decentralization of Gnutella, DHT uses a more structured routing method based on key–value pairs, as shown in Fig. 2.7. A structured network organizes all nodes in an orderly manner according to a certain structure. For example, Ethereum converts the public key of the node elliptic encryption algorithm into a NodeID with a length of 64 bytes as a unique identifier to distinguish nodes, so that Ethereum can achieve accurate node address search without a central server.

As shown in the Fig. 2.8, there are multiple super nodes in the hybrid network to form a distributed network, and each super node has multiple ordinary nodes and it forms a local centralized network. When a new ordinary node joins, first a super node is selected for communication and pushes the list of other super nodes to the newly joined node, while the joining node decides which specific super node to select as the parent node according to the super node status in the list. In practical applications, the hybrid structure is a relatively flexible and effective networking architecture, and the implementation difficulty is relatively small. Therefore, many systems are currently developed and implemented based on the hybrid structure.

2.3 Blockchain-Based AI System Framework

At present, with the rapid development of the both major technologies of blockchain and AI, more and more people have begun to compare the two to discuss the possibility of the integration and development of blockchain and AI. So, is it feasible to combine blockchain and AI? What are the advantages? This section will describe this in detail.

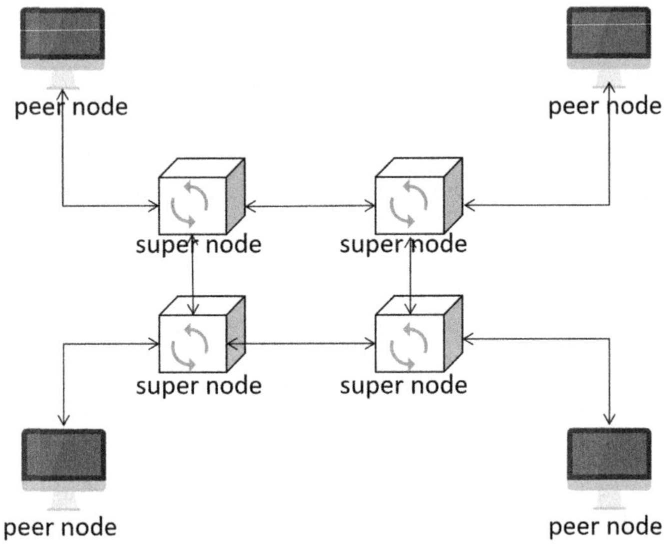

Fig. 2.8 Hybrid network structure

First of all, the research and application of blockchain and AI technology are based on a large amount of real data. As a distributed database, blockchain needs to ensure that multiple nodes in the network share real transaction records to form redundant backups, thereby ensuring the integrity and consistency of data on the chain. The development of AI algorithms also requires a large number of real training datasets. The more data collected, the more accurate the results of AI algorithms will be.

Second, blockchain technology can help AI applications to better improve the collection, storage and processing of data.

- In terms of data collection, the development of AI technology relies on a large amount of data. However, because the current data trading market is not yet developed, it is difficult for many small and medium-sized AI enterprises to obtain data. Blockchain aims to solve this problem by introducing peer-to-peer connections. Since it is an open distributed registry, everyone on the network can access the data. This will solve the problem of lack of algorithm training data caused by data oligopoly for many small and medium AI enterprises. Simultaneously, the difficulty of tampering with blockchain data also ensures the authenticity of the data.
- In terms of data storage and processing, the distributed data storage method of blockchain can improve the current centralized data storage and operation mode into a decentralized mode. Therefore, it is helpful to use distributed computing power to process data and speed up the training of AI algorithms.
- In terms of the standardizing and sharing of AI algorithms, each company in the industry currently has a self-sufficient set of AI algorithms, which makes it difficult to achieve interoperability between different applications. When the value chain

characteristics of the blockchain are used, firstly, the problem of paid sharing of algorithms can be solved to avoid infringement of intellectual property rights; secondly, enterprises can encapsulate AI services (data and algorithm codes) into API interfaces, which can be placed on the blockchain for other enterprises to pay for a fee, and the blockchain is responsible for registering and encrypting the corresponding data and algorithms, so it can help the AI market become more open and enable enterprises in the industry to cooperate easily.

Finally, AI will make the blockchain more autonomous and intelligent. The introduction of AI algorithms can improve the consensus mechanism of the blockchain and help humans make judgments through AI, such as intelligent voting and PoW computing power. In addition, the introduction of AI can also improve blockchain smart contracts, making the blockchain more intelligent.

If AI is a kind of productivity, it can improve the production efficiency and enable humans to obtain more wealth faster and more efficiently, then the blockchain is a production relationship. AI and blockchain can complement each other based on their respective strengths.

Figure 2.9 shows the technical application architecture of blockchain-integrated AI. The application of blockchain-integrated AI is based on data, algorithms and computing power. First of all, under the value of the blockchain and the difficulty to be tampered, the functions of data encryption, pricing, evaluation and transaction are realized in the data layer to build trusted data. Secondly, based on trusted data, the intelligent algorithm layer realizes the disassembly and invocation of AI algorithms, and the sharing of general intelligent algorithms, so as to disassemble the large-scale AI algorithms into multiple small tasks for different nodes. The individual intelligence of many nodes in the blockchain is integrated to realize group intelligence, and common algorithms are shared to avoid repeated work by each node. Finally, on the basis of trusted data and high-quality algorithms, the integrated application of AI and blockchain is completed. In this process, the sharing of blockchain computing power helps to solve the problem of insufficient computing power faced by the AI industry. The intelligent optimization of mining computing power aims to solve the problem of time and computing power consumption through research and development algorithms. Smart consensus and smart contracts are the introduction of AI to further improve the work efficiency of the blockchain.

2.4 Application of Blockchain and Artificial Intelligence in Healthcare

Now, there are several uses for blockchain and AI technology in the healthcare industry, including intelligent sharing of electronic medical records, intelligent prescription sharing, medical intelligence rating and traceability of drugs. The integration of blockchain and AI technology can effectively help to arrive at a diagnosis and enhance operational healthcare workflow. In the following sections, top uses of blockchain and AI in the healthcare sector will be introduced.

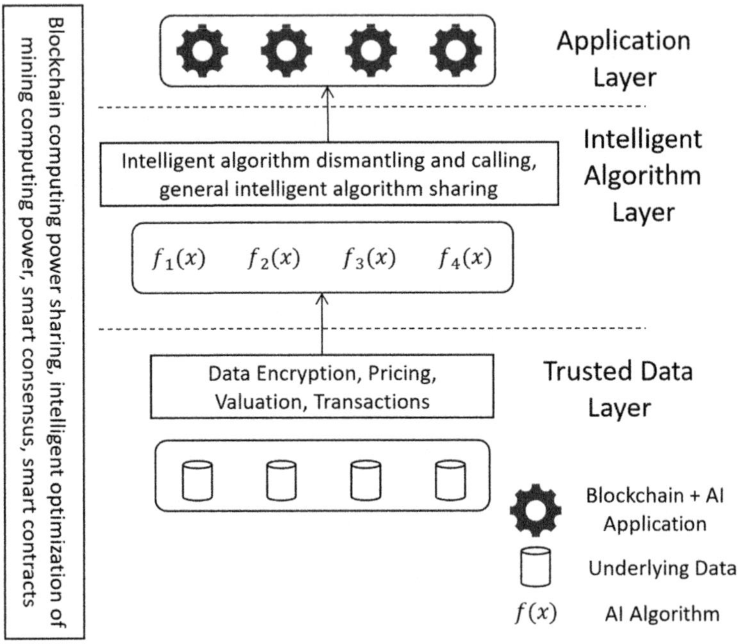

Fig. 2.9 Blockchain and AI fusion technology framework

2.4.1 Intelligent Sharing of Electronic Medical Records

In terms of intelligent medical care, a sharing platform for personal electronic medical records can be realized through blockchain technology. If medical records are imagined as a ledger, the blockchain can share the medical records originally in the various hospitals, patients can obtain their own medical records and historical conditions, and doctors can learn about the patients' medical historical record in details through the sharing platform. The shared platform establishes personal medical historical data for patients. Whether it is medical treatment or personal health planning, they can learn their physical condition and medical history through the shared medical record platform. The medical record data are completely taken charge by the patients themselves, not by a hospital or a third-party institution. The encryption mechanism of blockchain technology can also ensure that the sharing platform takes into account the privacy of patients and the security of medical record data. Patients can control their medical records to be open to any party and can also control the flow direction of medical records. The process of electronic medical records sharing is shown in Fig. 2.10.

In addition, the massive data of the blockchain can be used to make a health portrait of the individual, and the personal health model can regularly prompt the physical examination and balance the diet. Also, combined with the cure status in the electronic case database, different patients can get recommended hospitals or even

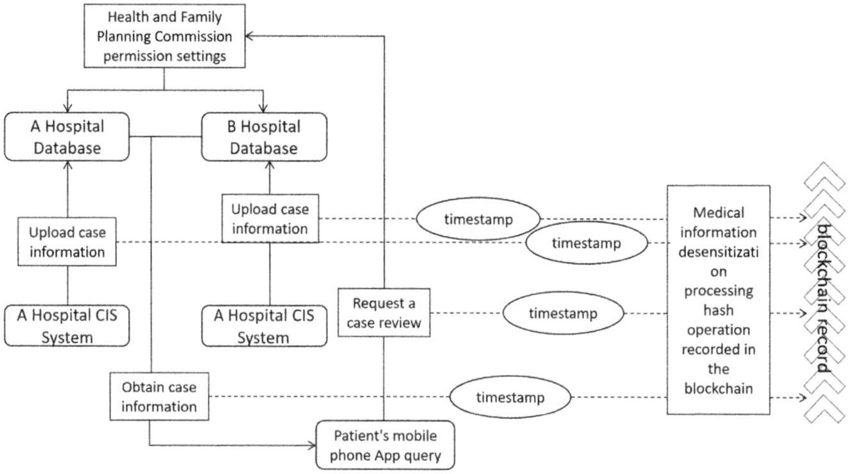

Fig. 2.10 Process of electronic medical records sharing

doctors in the smart electronic case. Through intelligent electronic medical records, preventive medical advice can be provided to patients based on their past medical history.

2.4.2 Intelligent Prescription Sharing

Intelligent prescription sharing means that doctors can view prescription information of similar conditions through the intelligent prescription sharing platform in the process of treating patients, so as to achieve the prescription sharing. At present, there are several problems in medical prescriptions, for example, patients modify prescriptions, doctors indiscriminately prescribe prescriptions; pharmacies and hospitals are separated, and the distribution process is opaque; the extreme imbalance of medical conditions leads to the inexperience of medical personnel in relatively poor areas, which delays patients' illness.

An intelligent prescription sharing platform based on blockchain technology can trace the origin of prescriptions while ensuring that patients do not tamper with prescriptions. Incorporating pharmacies into the blockchain platform network can effectively ensure the transparency and openness of drug distribution. The most important thing is that the sharing platform is conducive to improving the medical level of underdeveloped areas, and benefiting patients. Especially in remote areas in central and western China, patients can obtain prescriptions issued by major hospitals for different conditions through the prescription sharing platform, so as to obtain timely treatment advice. The framework of the intelligent prescription sharing platform is shown in Fig. 2.11.

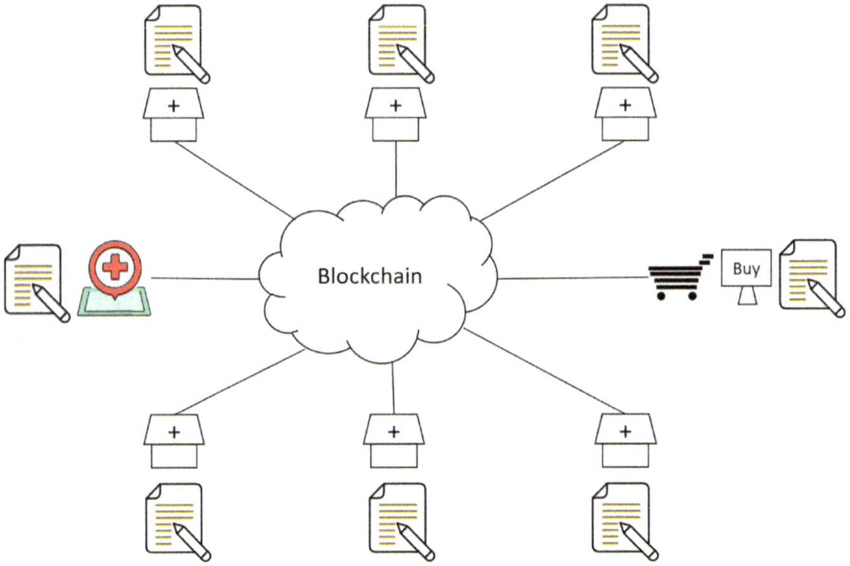

Fig. 2.11 Intelligent prescription sharing platform framework

The blockchain technology is used to realize the connection between hospitals and cooperative pharmacies, establish a quasi-real-time prescription distribution mechanism and ensure the consistency and integrity of prescriptions between hospitals and pharmacies. Each prescription has a prescription label, and the platform strictly controls the repeated use of prescriptions. When the same prescription label appears, the entire network will be notified for verification to prevent the chaos of prescription reuse.

2.4.3 *Medical Intelligence Rating*

Medical intelligence rating refers to the establishment of an alliance medical platform between regulatory authorities and major hospitals based on blockchain technology to supervise the cases and prescriptions of major hospitals across the country, effectively shorten the query repetition cycle, and ensure data integrity and transparency. In addition, the intelligent rating system will also establish a medical rating model with the data of each hospital in the blockchain, and regularly rate the Class A tertiary hospitals, which can effectively prevent the hospitals from acting independently and help improve the comprehensive medical strength.

2.4.4 *Traceability of Drugs*

The integration of blockchain technology and Internet of Things technology can realize the traceability of the entire cycle of drugs. The Internet of Things technology is used to collect and monitor data during the procurement and transportation of pharmaceutical raw materials, which are input into the blockchain distributed database for tracking. In the process of drug production and manufacturing, real-time surveillance and evaluation of production and sale data can be realized by opening up the data channel of the manufacturing execution systems (EMS), enterprise resource planning (ERP) and blockchain traceability system. The drug traceability system has supervision nodes, all produced drugs need to be signed by the digital certificate of the regulatory node before they can enter the market. On the application side, traceability media such as user App, QR code, WeChat applet, etc. can be provided, so that users can flexibly and conveniently trace the whole process data of drugs.

Chapter 3
Medical Imaging

3.1 Introduction

In this book, a kind of signal and system approach is taken to the characterization of medical imaging. In practice, the patients' signals with various diseases are transformed into images via medical imaging modalities, and the signal of interest is defined by the modality and specific imaging parameters. These signals arise from four processes:

- Transmission of x-rays through the body (in projection radiography and CT).
- Emission of gamma rays from radiotracers in the body (in nuclear medicine).
- Reflection of ultrasonic waves within the body (in ultrasound imaging).
- Precession of spin systems in a large magnetic field (in MRI).

The medical imaging areas we consider in details in this book are projection radiography, CT, nuclear medicine, ultrasound imaging and MRI. An *imaging modality* is a particular imaging technique or system within one of these areas. In this section, we give a brief overview of these most common imaging modalities.

Projection radiography uses ionizing radiation, which is termed transmission imaging modalities. It includes routine diagnostic radiography, digital radiography, angiography, neuroradiology, mobile x-ray systems and mammography. All of these modalities are called "projection" radiography because they all represent the projection of a 3D object or signal onto a 2D image. It transmits x-rays through the body, then uses the fact that the body's tissues selectively attenuate the x-ray intensities to form an image. Shadows have been created by dense objects (such as bone) in the body. This intensity distribution is revealed using a scintillator, which converts the x-rays to visible light. Finally, the light image on the scintillator is captured either on a large sheet of photographic film, a camera, or solid-state detectors. A property of projection radiographic methods is that structures located at different depths in the body are overlaid (or superimposed) on the 2D image.

S. Guo et al., *Advanced Technologies in Healthcare*,
https://doi.org/10.1007/978-981-99-9585-1_3

As in projection radiography, *Computed Tomography* uses x-rays. Unlike projection radiography, CT collects multiple projections of the same tissues from different orientations by moving the x-ray source around the body. CT systems have rows of digital detectors whose signals are input directly to a computer, and these signals are used to reconstruct one or more cross sections (slices) of the human body. In this way, CT systems generate truly tomographic images after reconstruction. CT includes the following modalities:

- *Single-slice CT*, which acquires data within a single plane and reconstructs only one plane per rotation.
- *Helical CT*, the x-ray tube and detectors continuously rotate around in a large circle, while the patient is moved in a continuous motion through the circle's center (acquire 3D data in less than a minute).
- *Multiple-row detector CT*, there are many rows of detectors used to rapidly gather a cone of x-ray data.

Nuclear medicine uses ionizing radiation, which is emission imaging modalities. In nuclear medicine, radioactive compounds are injected into the body. The molecules of these substances are labeled with radionuclides that emit gamma rays. These compounds or tracers move selectively to different regions or organs within the body, emitting gamma rays with intensity proportional to the compound's local concentration. A nuclear medicine image reflects the local concentration of a radiotracer within the body. There are three modalities within nuclear medicine: *conventional radionuclide imaging or scintigraphy*, *single-photon emission CT (SPECT)* and *positron emission tomography (PET)*. Conventional radionuclide imaging and SPECT typically utilize a special 2D gamma ray scintillation detector called an Anger camera, which is designed to detect single x-rays or gamma rays. In conventional radionuclide imaging, this procedure combines the effects of emission with the effects of attenuation of the rays by intervening body tissues, producing images that are 2D projections of the 3D distribution of radiotracers confounded by attenuation. SPECT and PET produce images of slices within the body. SPECT does this by rotating the Anger camera around the body. In PET, a radionuclide decay produces a positron, which immediately annihilates to produce two gamma rays flying off in opposite directions. The PET scanner looks for coincident detections from opposing detectors in its ring, thus determining the line that passes through the site where the annihilation occurred. Both SPECT and PET use computed tomography reconstruction techniques including iterative reconstruction in order to create diagnostic images.

Ultrasound imaging is often called reflection imaging. Ultrasound imaging uses electrical-to-acoustical transducers to generate repetitive bursts of high-frequency sound. These pulses travel into the soft tissue of the body and reflect back to the transducer. The time-of-return of these pulses gives information about the location of a reflector, and the intensity of these pulses gives information about the strength of a reflector. By rapidly moving or scanning the transducer or its acoustical beam, real-time images of cross sections of soft tissue can be generated. They are designed primarily to image anatomy, which are comparatively inexpensive and completely noninvasive. Ultrasound imaging systems offer several imaging modalities:

- *A-mode imaging*, which generates a one-dimensional waveform, and as such does not really comprise an image. This mode can provide very detailed information about rapid or subtle motion.
- *B-mode imaging*, which is ordinary cross-sectional anatomical imaging.
- *M-mode imaging* generates a series of A-mode signals, which are modulated by brightness and displayed in real-time on a computer display. It is important for measuring the time-varying displacement of a heart valve.
- *Doppler imaging*, which uses the property of frequency or phase shift caused by moving objects to generate images that are color coded by their motion, is most commonly used in an audio mode.
- *Nonlinear imaging*, which permits higher resolution imaging at greater depths.
- *Magnetic resonance* scanners use the property of nuclear magnetic resonance to create images. MRI requires a combination of a high-strength magnetic field and radio frequency Faraday induction to image properties of the proton nucleus of the hydrogen atom. MRI includes the following modalities:
- *Standard MRI*, which includes a whole host of pulse sequences.
- *Echo-planar imaging* (EPI).
- *Magnetic resonance spectroscopic imaging* (MRS), which records images of other nuclei besides that of the hydrogen atom.
- *Functional MRI* (fMRI), which uses oxygenation-sensitive pulse sequences to image blood oxygenation in the brain.
- *Diffusion MRI* (dMRI), which images the degree and orientation of molecular diffusion in tissue.

Different medical imaging modalities reveal different properties of the human body. As a result, it is often useful to obtain diagnostic images of a single patient and medical condition using multiple modalities. Combining CT and PET is particularly useful because PET provides functional information that complements the structural information provided by CT and also because the CT data can be directly used to improve the reconstructed PET images.

3.2 Image Formation

In this section, the mathematical models are developed to characterize image formation using projection radiography as an example.

Fig. 3.1 The geometry of a conventional projection radiographic system

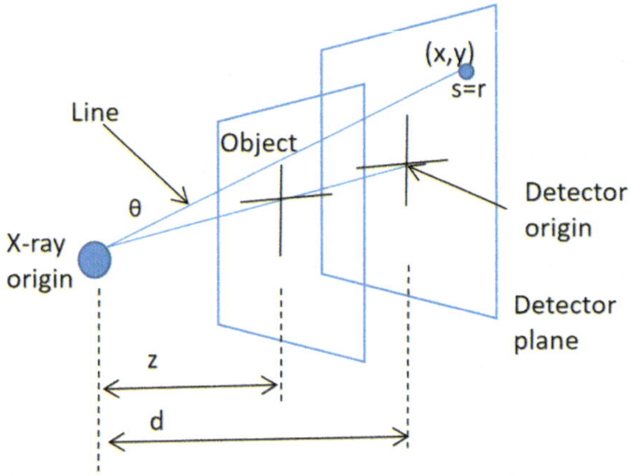

3.2.1 Basic Imaging Equation

The x-ray tube emits a burst of x-rays that, after filtration and restriction, are incident upon the patient. These x-rays are then attenuated as they pass through the body in a spatial pattern that depends on the linear attenuation coefficient distribution in the body. Consider a particular line segment through the object starting at the x-ray origin and ending on the detector plane at point (x, y), as shown in Fig. 3.1. The linear attenuation is a function of x, y and z, in general; on the line, it can be considered to be a function of its distance s from the origin. Suppose that the length of the line segment is $r = r(x, y)$, the intensity of x-rays incident on the detector at (x, y) is given by

$$I(x, y) = \int_0^{E_{\max}} S_0(E')E'\exp\left\{-\int_0^{r(x,y)} \mu(s; E', x, y)ds\right\}dE', \tag{3.1}$$

where $S_0(E)$ is the spectrum of the incident x-rays. Any photon "survives" its passage through the body then hits the detector apparatus, and is either absorbed by the detector itself, or exits out the back of the detector.

3.2.2 Geometric Effects

X-ray images are created from a diverging beam of x-rays; this divergence produces a number of undesirable effects that arise from geometric considerations. These effects are multiplicative, which are demonstrated as follows.

Inverse Square Law. The inverse square law states that the net flux of photons decreases as $1/r^2$, where r is the distance from the x-ray origin. Assume that the beam intensity integrated over a small sphere surrounding the source is given by I_S.

Let the source-to-detector distance be d. Assuming there is no object causing beam attenuation between the source and the detector, the intensity at the origin of the detector is

$$I_0 = \frac{I_s}{4\pi d^2}. \tag{3.2}$$

The intensity at an arbitrary point (x, y) on the detector is smaller than that at the detector origin simply because it is farther away from the x-ray source. Let $r = r(x, y)$ be the distance between the x-ray origin and the detector point (x, y). Then the intensity at (x, y) is

$$I_r = \frac{I_s}{4\pi r^2}, \tag{3.3}$$

$$I_r = I_0 \frac{d^2}{r^2} = I_0 cos^2\theta. \tag{3.4}$$

Thus, the inverse square law causes a $\cos^2\theta$ drop-off of x-ray intensity away from the detector origin, even without object attenuation.

Obliquity. Obliquity is a second factor that acts to decrease the beam intensity away from the detector origin. The obliquity effect is caused by the detector surface not being orthogonal to the direction of x-ray propagation. This fact implies that x-rays passing through a unit area orthogonal to the direction of x-ray propagation actually pass through a larger area on the detector. Thus, the x-ray flux is lower, which directly results in a lower measured x-ray intensity on the detector surface. Given an area A orthogonal to the direction of x-ray propagation, the projected area on the detector is $A_d = A/\cos\theta$. Therefore, the measured intensity due to obliquity alone is

$$I_d = I_0 \cos\theta. \tag{3.5}$$

Beam Divergence and Flat Detector. The effects of beam divergence and the flat detector act together to reduce intensity at the detector plane in two ways: (1) reduction in beam intensity due to the inverse square law effect and (2) reduction in beam intensity due to obliquity. The combination of these two effects is multiplicative. So, the overall beam intensity relative to the intensity I_0 at the detector origin, assuming no object attenuation, is given by

$$I_d(x, y) = I_0 \cos^3\theta. \tag{3.6}$$

Anode Heel Effect. The reason for the anode heel effect is due to the geometry of the anode, and the anode heel effect far outweighs the effects of obliquity and inverse square law in its overall effect on the uniformity of intensity across the detector surface. The anode heel effect can be compensated by using an x-ray filter that is

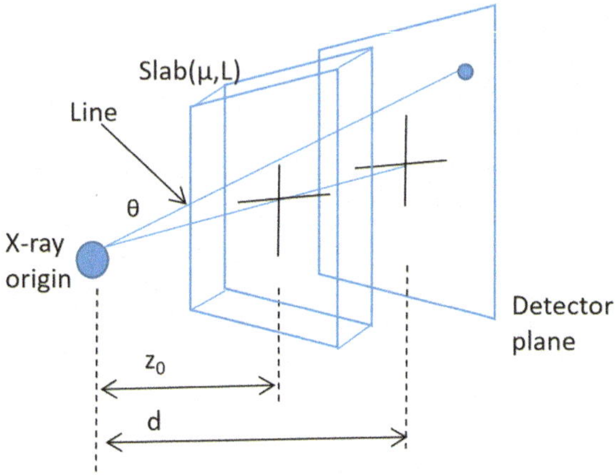

Fig. 3.2 Imaging a uniform slab

thicker in the cathode direction than in the anode direction. In particular, the anode heel effect should be used as a kind of inherent compensation for natural gradients in the body's x-ray attenuation profile. In the development of x-ray imaging equations, assume that the anode heel effect is compensated by filtration.

Path Length. Consider imaging a slab of material with a constant linear attenuation coefficient μ and thickness L arranged parallel to the plane of the detector, as shown in Fig. 3.2. The central ray of the x-ray beam encounters a net path length L through the object. Thus, the x-ray intensity at $(x, y) = (0, 0)$ will be $I_0\exp(-\mu L)$, where I_0 is the intensity of the beam that would be present at the detector origin if the slab were not present.

If the inverse square law and obliquity are included, then the intensity is given by

$$I_d(x, y) = I_0 \cos^3 \theta e^{-\mu L/\cos\theta}. \tag{3.7}$$

If the anode heel effect is compensated by filtration, then this equation represents a valid imaging equation for a homogeneous slab parallel to the image plane within the field of view.

Depth-Dependent Magnification. Another consequence of divergent x-rays is object magnification, which is specifically called depth-dependent magnification in radiography. It is clear from the geometry that the object will always appear larger on the detector than it is in reality. Using the concept of similar triangles, it is easy to show that when the object is at position z, its height w_z on the detector will be

$$w_z = w\frac{d}{z}. \tag{3.8}$$

And the magnification $M(z)$ is given by

$$M(z) = \frac{d}{z}. \tag{3.9}$$

Imaging Equation with Geometric Effects. An idealized object $t_z(x, y)$ is utilized that is infinitesimally thin and located in a single plane given by the coordinate z and is capable of differentially attenuating x-rays as a function of x and y. If the object is located at the detector face, the recorded intensity would be

$$I_d(x, y) = I_0 \cos^3 \theta t_d(x, y), \tag{3.10}$$

where

$$\cos\theta = \frac{d}{\sqrt{d^2 + x^2 + y^2}}. \tag{3.11}$$

In general, when the object is located at arbitrary z, the magnification must be taken into account and it is

$$I_d(x, y) = I_0 \left(\frac{d}{\sqrt{d^2 + x^2 + y^2}} \right)^3 t_z(xz/d, yz/d). \tag{3.12}$$

3.2.3 Blurring Effects

There are two effects that will blur objects: extended sources and the detector thickness. Both of these processes can be modeled as convolutional effects that degrade image resolution. These two effects are shown in details.

Extended Sources. It is clear that the extended source effect is a convolution of the source shape with the object shape. Because of this, extended sources produce a significant loss of resolution of x-ray images. The physical extent of blurring caused by extended sources depends on the size of the source spot and the location of the object. Consider the image of the point hole shown in Fig. 3.3. From the geometry, if the source has diameter D, then the image of the point hole located at range z will have diameter D', given by

$$D' = \frac{d - z}{z} D. \tag{3.13}$$

The source magnification $m(z)$ is given by

$$m(z) = -\frac{d - z}{z}. \tag{3.14}$$

It can be seen that the depth-dependent magnification and the source magnification are related as $m(z) = 1 - M(z)$.

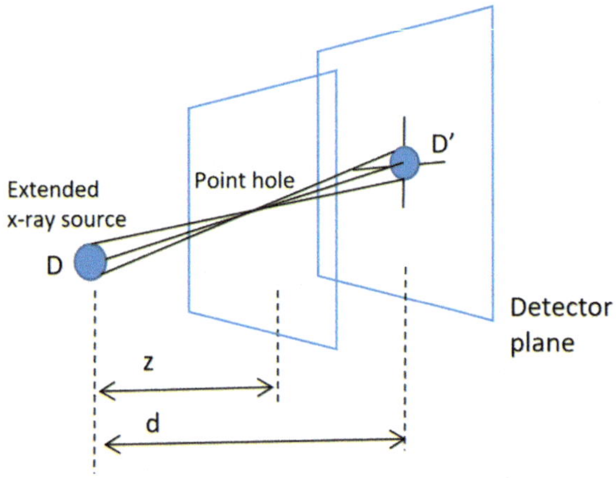

Fig. 3.3 Principle of source magnification

To develop an imaging equation incorporating source magnification, the image of the point hole on the z-axis is considered. Let the x-ray tube source spot be represented by the source intensity distribution $s(x, y)$, and ignoring geometric effects, the intensity distribution is

$$I_d(x, y) = ks(x/m, y/m), \tag{3.15}$$

where m is the source magnification for a point at range z. The amplitude scaling term k must be found. The integrated intensity on the detector plane must remain constant, which implies that

$$k \propto \frac{1}{m^2(z)}. \tag{3.16}$$

Then the superposition is used to understand the behavior of a spatial distribution of attenuating objects within a given z plane, which leads to an imaging equation that is the convolution of the magnified object by the magnified and scaled source function,

$$I_d(x, y) = \frac{\cos^3\theta}{4\pi d^2 m^2} s(x/m, y/m) * t_z(x/M, y/M). \tag{3.17}$$

Film-Screen and Digital Detector Blurring. For each x-ray photon that is absorbed by a phosphor, a large number of lower-energy light photons are produced. The light photons travel isotropically from the point where the x-ray is absorbed, and they can then be absorbed in the film at locations far from the x-ray's path. The union of detected light photons form a "spot" on the film, which is effectively an impulse response to the x-ray "impulse". Using superposition, an imaging equation incorporating film-screen blurring is readily derived.

$$I_d(x, y) = \frac{\cos^3 \theta}{4\pi d^2 m^2} s(x/m, y/m) * t_z(x/M, y/M) * h(x, y). \tag{3.18}$$

3.3 Image Quality

3.3.1 *Introduction*

The primary purpose of a medical imaging system is to create images of the internal structures and functions of the human body that can be used by medical professionals to diagnose abnormal conditions, determine the underlying mechanisms that produce and control these conditions, guide therapeutic procedures and monitor the effectiveness of treatment. The ability of medical professionals to successfully accomplish these tasks strongly depends on the quality of the images acquired by the medical imaging system at hand. Image quality depends on the particular used imaging modality. This task is simplified by focusing on the following six important factors: (1) contrast, (2) resolution, (3) noise, (4) artifacts, (5) distortion and (6) accuracy.

The ability of medical professionals to discriminate among anatomical or functional features in a given image strongly depends on *contrast*. Contrast quantifies the difference between image characteristics of an object and surrounding objects or background. High contrast allows easier identification of individual objects in an image, whereas low contrast makes this task difficult.

The ability of a medical imaging system to depict details is known as *resolution*. High resolution systems create images of high diagnostic quality. Low resolution systems create images that lack fine detail.

A medical image may be corrupted by random fluctuations in image intensity that do not contribute to image quality. It is known as *noise*. The source, amount and type of noise depends on the particular used imaging modality. Object visibility is often reduced by the presence of noise, because the noise masks image features.

Most medical imaging systems can create image features that do not represent a valid object within, or characteristic of, the patient. These features are known as *artifacts*, and can frequently obscure important features or be falsely interpreted as abnormal findings.

Medical images should not only make desired features visible but should also give an accurate impression of their shape, size, position and other geometric characteristics. Unfortunately, for many reasons, medical imaging systems frequently introduce *distortion* of these important factors. Distortion in medical images should be corrected in order to improve the diagnostic quality of these images.

Fundamentally, the *accuracy* of medical images is interested in the context of a clinical application, where "accuracy" means both conformity to truth and clinical utility.

Table 3.1 The way to characterize factors which affect the quality of medical image

	The way to characterize factors
Contrast	Modulation, modulation transfer function, local contrast
Resolution	Line spread function, full width at half maximum, modulation transfer function, resolution tool
Noise	Random variables, signal-to-noise ratio
Artifacts and distortion	Motion artifact, star artifact, ring artifact, etc. size distortion, shape distortion
Accuracy	Quantitative accuracy: bias, imprecision diagnostic accuracy: sensitivity, specificity

Table 3.1 shows the main way to characterize factors which affect the quality of medical image.

3.3.2 Contrast

In general, the goal of a medical imaging system is to accurately portray or preserve the true object contrast in the image. Particularly for detection of abnormalities, a medical imaging system that produces high contrast images is preferable to a system that produces low contrast images, since anatomical and functional features are easier to identify in high contrast images.

Modulation: Using of a periodic signal and its modulation is an effective way to quantify contrast. The modulation m_f of a periodic signal $f(x, y)$ is defined by

$$m_f = \frac{f_{\max} - f_{\min}}{f_{\max} + f_{\min}} \tag{3.19}$$

where m_f refers to the contrast of the periodic signal $f(x, y)$ relative to its average value. In practice, the usual presence of a nonzero "background" intensity in a medical image reduces image contrast. If $m_f = 0$, it can be said that $f(x, y)$ has no contrast. If f(x, y) and g(x, y) are two periodic signals with the same average value, it can be said that $f(x, y)$ has more contrast than $g(x, y)$ if $m_f > m_g$.

Modulation Transfer Function: The way that a medical imaging system affects contrast can be investigated by imaging a sinusoidal object $f(x, y)$ of the form $f(x, y) = A + B\sin(2\pi u_0 x)$, so the modulation of $f(x, y)$ is given by

$$m_f = \frac{B}{A}. \tag{3.20}$$

The output $g(x, y)$ of the system is given by $g(x, y) = AH(0, 0) + B|H(u_0, 0)|\sin(2\pi u_0 x)$, in which case the modulation of $g(x, y)$ is given by

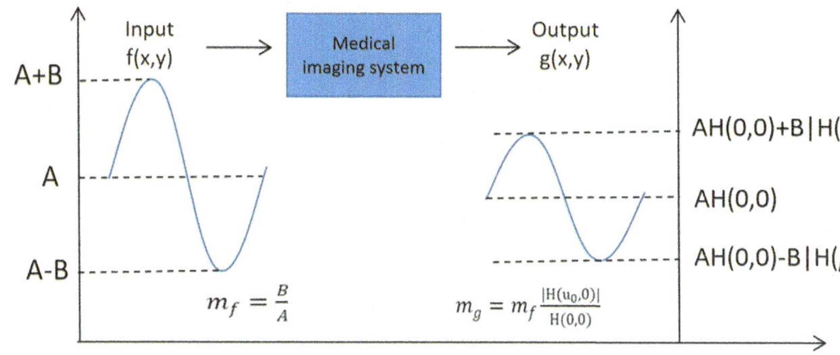

Fig. 3.4 Basic principles for determining the modulation of the output of a medical imaging system from the modulation of the input, when the input object is sinusoidal

$$m_g = m_f \frac{|H(u_0, 0)|}{H(0, 0)}. \tag{3.21}$$

The ratio of the output modulation to the input modulation as a function of spatial frequency is called the modulation transfer function (MTF), and is given by

$$\text{MTF}(u) = \frac{m_g}{m_f} = \frac{|H(u, 0)|}{H(0, 0)} \tag{3.22}$$

This shows that the MTF of a medical imaging system is the "frequency response" of the system. Because of the way that a medical imaging system affects modulation, the contrast, is illustrated in Fig. 3.4.

Local Contrast: The identification of some specific object or feature within an image is only possible if its value differs from that of surrounding areas. It is common in many imaging modalities to refer to an object of interest as the target, as illustrated in Fig. 3.5. The target is surrounded by other issues, called the background. Suppose that the target has a nominal image intensity of f_t and the background has a nominal image intensity of f_b. The difference between the target and its background is captured by the local contrast, defined as

$$C = \frac{f_t - f_b}{f_b} \tag{3.23}$$

3.3.3 Resolution

Resolution can be thought of as the ability of a medical imaging system to accurately depict two distinct events in space, time, or frequency as separation. Resolution can also be thought of as the degree of smearing, or blurring, when a medical imaging

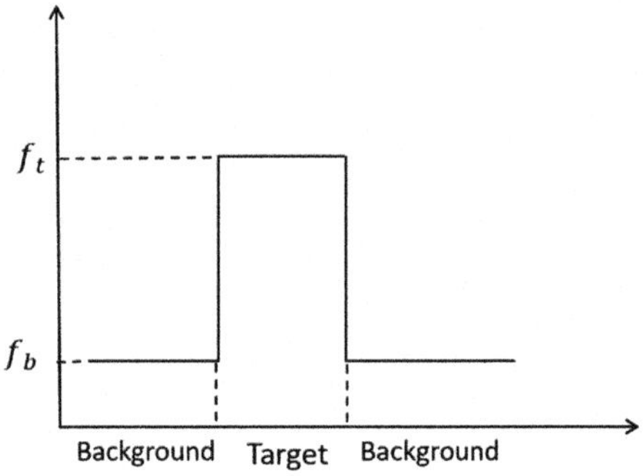

Fig. 3.5 Local contrast scenario

system is introduces to a single event in space, time, or frequency. These two ways of looking at resolution are related, and a high resolution medical imaging system is characterized by low smearing, whereas a low resolution system is characterized by high smearing.

Line Spread Function: The traditional point spread function (PSF), the response of an imaging system to a point source is often used to characterize resolution. As an alternative, it can be considered that the response of a medical imaging system to a line impulse. This line source can be mathematically represented by the line impulse, since the system is isotropic, shown as $f(x, y) = \delta(x)$. Then the output $g(x, y)$ of the system will be given by

$$g(x, y) = \int_{-\infty}^{\infty}\int_{-\infty}^{\infty} h(\xi, \eta)\delta(x - \xi)d\xi d\eta = \int_{-\infty}^{\infty} h(x, \eta)d\eta \tag{3.24}$$

The resulting image $g(x, y)$ is only a function of x, which is known as the line spread function (LSF) of the system, and can be used to quantify resolution.

Full Width at Half Maximum: Given the LSF of a medical imaging system, its resolution can be quantified using a measure called the full width at half maximum (FWHM). This is the width of the LSF at one-half its maximum value. The FWHM equals the minimum distance that two lines must be separated in space in order to appear as separateness in the recorded image, which is depicted in Fig. 3.6. A decrease in the FWHM indicates an improvement in resolution.

Resolution and Modulation Transfer Function: Another way to quantify the resolution of a medical imaging system is as the smallest separation between two adjacent maxima in a sinusoidal input that can be resolved in the image. Consider the input of a medical imaging system is $f(x, y) = B\sin(2\pi ux)$, the output of the system is given by $g(x, y) = \text{MTF}(u)H(0, 0)B\sin(2\pi ux)$. Notice that the separation between two adjacent maxima of the sinusoidal input $f(x, y)$ is $1/u$. The recorded image $g(x, y)$ is also sinusoidal, with $1/u$ being the separation between two adjacent maxima as well. For some spatial cutoff frequency u_c, in which case, $g(x, y) = 0$ for every $u > u_c$, and the resolution of the system will be $1/u_c$. The MTF can be

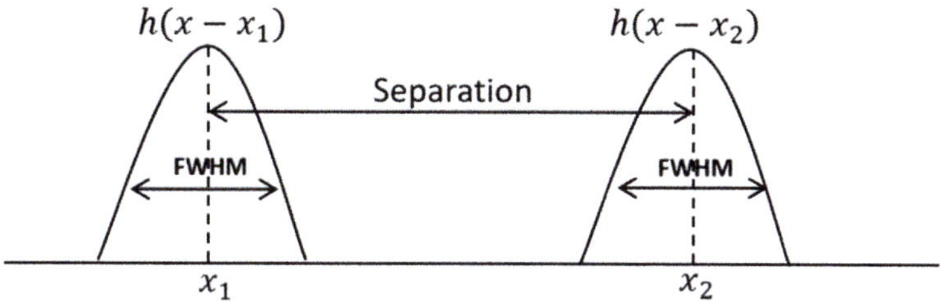

Fig. 3.6 An example of the effect of system resolution on the ability to differentiate two points (The FWHM equals the minimum distance that the two points must be separated in order to be distinguishable)

directly obtained from the LSF,

$$\mathrm{MTF}(u) = \frac{|L(u)|}{L(0)}. \tag{3.25}$$

Therefore, the MTF equals the (normalized) magnitude of the 1D Fourier transform of the LSF.

From the above discussion, it can be found that the MTF can be effectively used to compare two competing medical imaging systems in terms of their contrast and resolution. If the MTFs of the two systems under consideration are of a similar shape but have a different cutoff frequency, it can be concluded that the system with higher MTF values will be better in terms of contrast and resolution. If the MTF curves are of different shapes, the situation is more complicated. In Fig. 3.7, SYSTEM 1 has better low-frequency contrast, and is thus better for imaging coarse details, while SYSTEM 2 has a better high-frequency contrast, and is thus better for imaging fine details. The FWHM of the PSF or LSF is the most direct metric of resolution.

Subsystem Cascade: Medical imaging systems are often modeled as a cascade of linear shift-invariant (LSI) subsystems, the recorded image $g(x, y)$ can be modeled as the convolution of the input object $f(x, y)$ with the PSF of the first subsystem, followed by the convolution with the PSF of the second subsystem, etc., shown in the formula (3.26).

Fig. 3.7 MTF curves of two competing medical imaging systems

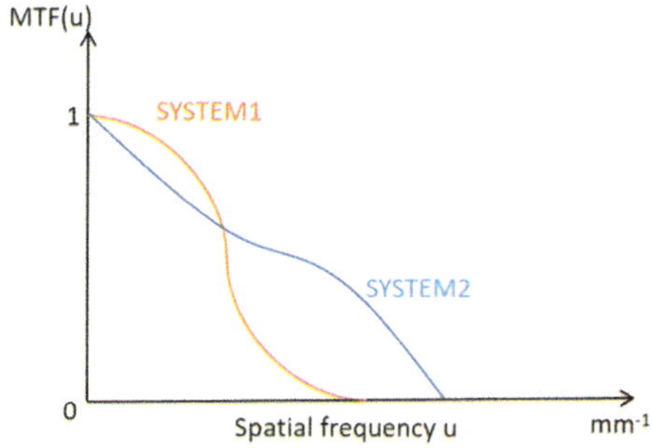

$$g(x, y) = h_k(x, y)*\cdots*(h_2(x, y)*(h_1(x, y)*f(x, y))). \tag{3.26}$$

If the resolution is quantified using the FWHM, then the FWHM of the overall system can be determined approximately from the FWHMs $R_1, R_2, \cdots, R_k$ of the individual subsystems, by

$$R = \sqrt{R_1^2 + R_2^2 + \cdots R_k^2}. \tag{3.27}$$

If contrast and resolution are quantified using the MTF, then the MTF of the overall system will be given by

$$\text{MTF}(u, v) = \text{MTF}_1(u, v)\text{MTF}_2(u, v)\cdots\text{MTF}_k(u, v) \tag{3.28}$$

and its frequency response $H(u, v)$ of the overall system is given by

$$H(u, v) = H_1(u, v)H_2(u, v)\cdots H_k(u, v). \tag{3.29}$$

If one subsystem has a small value of the MTF at some spatial frequency, then the MTF of the overall system will be small at that frequency as well. In other words, the MTF of the overall system will always be less than the MTF of each subsystem. Therefore, the overall quality of a medical imaging system, in terms of contrast and resolution, will be inferior to the quality of each subsystem.

Resolution Tool: Resolution can be quantified in terms of the ability of a system to image details of a given test pattern. For example, one common way to measure resolution for a particular system is to image the so-called resolution tool or bar phantom, which is composed of groups of parallel lines of a certain width, separated by gaps having the same width as the line width. Each group is characterized by the density of such lines, and measured in line pairs per millimeter (l p/mm). The tool is imaged through the system under consideration, and system resolution is reported as the frequency (in lp/mm) of the finest line group that can be resolved at the output.

3.3.4 Noise

An unwanted characteristic of medical imaging system is noise. Image quality decreases as noise increases. A general way to characterize noise is to consider it as the numerical outcome of a random event or experiment.

Random Variables: The numerical quantity associated with a random event or experiment is called a random variable. It is mathematically described by $P_N(\eta)$, its probability distribution function (PDF), given by

$$P_N(\eta) = \Pr[N \leq \eta]. \tag{3.30}$$

where the PDF gives the probability that random variable N will take on a value less than or equal to η.

Continuous Random Variables: If $P_N(\eta)$ is a continuous function of η, then N is a continuous random variable. This random variable is uniquely specified by its probability density function,

$$p_N(\eta) = \frac{dP_N(\eta)}{d\eta} \tag{3.31}$$

which satisfies the following three properties:

$$p_N(\eta) \geq 0, \int_{-\infty}^{\infty} p_N(\eta)d\eta = 1, P_N(\eta) = \int_{-\infty}^{\infty} p_N(u)du. \tag{3.32}$$

A random variable is often characterized by its expected value(mean)

$$\mu_N = E[N] = \int_{-\infty}^{\infty} \eta p_N(\eta)d\eta \tag{3.33}$$

and its variance

$$\sigma_N^2 = Var[N] = E[(N - \mu_N)^2] = \int_{-\infty}^{\infty} (\eta - \mu_N)^2 p_N(\eta)d\eta. \tag{3.34}$$

Furthermore, the square root of the variance is called the standard deviation of N. The mean can be thought of as the average value of the random variable, whereas the standard deviation can be thought of as the "average" variation of the values of the random variable about its mean. The larger the standard deviation, the "more random" the random variable becomes.

Discrete Random Variables: This random variable is uniquely specified by the probability mass function (PMF) $\Pr[N = \eta_i]$.

Independent Random Variables: When the random variables are independent,

$$\mu_s = \mu_1 + \mu_2 + \cdots + \mu_m \tag{3.35}$$

$$\sigma_s^2 = \sigma_1^2 + \sigma_2^2 + \cdots + \sigma_m^2 \tag{3.36}$$

$$p_s(\eta) = p_1(\eta) * p_2(\eta) * \cdots * p_m(\eta). \tag{3.37}$$

3.3.5 Signal-To-Noise Ratio

It is assumed that the output of a medical imaging system is a random variable G, composed of two components, f and N. Component f, which is usually referred to as signal, is the "true" value of G, whereas N is a random fluctuation or error component due to noise. The identification of an abnormal condition within the human body most often depends on how "close" an observed value g of G is to its true value f. A useful way to quantify this is by means of the signal-to-noise ratio (SNR), which describes the relative "strength" of signal f with respect to that of noise N. Higher image quality requires that the output of a medical imaging system be characterized by high SNR. Blurring reduces contrast and thus SNR; noise also reduces SNR.

Amplitude SNR: The SNR is expressed as the ratio of signal amplitude to noise amplitude:

$$\mathrm{SNR}_a = \frac{\mathrm{Amplitude}(f)}{\mathrm{Amplitude}(N)}. \tag{3.38}$$

Power SNR: Another way to express the SNR is as the ratio of signal power to noise power:

$$\mathrm{SNR}_p = \frac{\mathrm{power}(f)}{\mathrm{power}(N)}. \tag{3.39}$$

If assuming that the noise mean and variance do not depend on (x, y) (a common assumption that characterizes so-called wide-sense stationary noise), then it can be shown that

$$\mathrm{SNR}_p = \frac{\int_{-\infty}^{\infty}\int_{-\infty}^{\infty}|h(x, y)*f(x, y)|^2 dxdy}{\int_{-\infty}^{\infty}\int_{-\infty}^{\infty}\mathrm{NPS}(u, v)dudv}, \tag{3.40}$$

$$\mathrm{NPS}(u, v) = \lim_{x_0, y_0 \to \infty} \frac{1}{4x_0 y_0} \mathrm{E}\left[\left|\int_{-x_0}^{x_0}\int_{-y_0}^{y_0}[N(x, y) - \mu_N]\exp(-j2\pi(ux + vy))dxdy\right|^2\right], \tag{3.41}$$

is known as the noise power spectrum (NPS). From Parseval's theorem, it has

$$\begin{aligned}\mathrm{SNR}_p &= \frac{\int_{-\infty}^{\infty}\int_{-\infty}^{\infty}|H(u, v)|^2|F(u, v)|^2 dudv}{\int_{-\infty}^{\infty}\int_{-\infty}^{\infty}\mathrm{NPS}(u, v)dudv} \\ &= \frac{\int_{-\infty}^{\infty}\int_{-\infty}^{\infty}\mathrm{SNR}_p(u, v)\mathrm{NPS}(u, v)dudv}{\int_{-\infty}^{\infty}\int_{-\infty}^{\infty}\mathrm{NPS}(u, v)dudv},\end{aligned} \tag{3.42}$$

where

$$\mathrm{SNR}_p(u,v) = \frac{|H(u,v)|^2|F(u,v)|^2}{\mathrm{NPS}(u,v)} = \frac{\mathrm{MTF}^2(u,v)}{\mathrm{NPS}(u,v)}|F(u,v)|^2 H^2(0,0) \quad (3.43)$$

is called the frequency-dependent power SNR. The frequency-dependent power SNR quantifies, at a given frequency, the relative "strength" of signal to that of noise at the output of the LSI system. $\mathrm{SNR}_p(u,v)$ provides a relationship among contrast, resolution, noise and image quality. For a given output noise level and a given input $f(x,y)$, better contrast and resolution properties (i.e., a larger MTF) result in better image quality (i.e., a higher output power SNR).

Differential SNR: Consider an object (or target) of interest placed on a background. Let f_t and f_b be the average image intensities within the target and background. A useful choice for SNR is obtained by taking the "signal" to be difference in average image intensity values between the target and the background integrated over the area A of the target, and by taking the "noise" to be the random fluctuation of image intensity from its mean over an area A of the background. It leads to the differential signal-to-noise ratio, given by

$$\mathrm{SNR}_{\mathrm{diff}} = \frac{A(f_t - f_b)}{\sigma_b(A)}, \quad (3.44)$$

where $\sigma_b(A)$ is the standard deviation of image intensity values from their mean over an area A of the background. It further has

$$\mathrm{SNR}_{\mathrm{diff}} = \frac{\mathrm{CAf}_b}{\sigma_b(A)} \quad (3.45)$$

which relates the differential SNR to contrast.

3.3.6 Artifacts and Distortion

Artifacts can obscure important targets, and they can be falsely interpreted as valid image features. Moreover, they can impair correct detection and characterization of features of interest by adding "clutter" to images. Evaluation and possibly removal of artifacts should be part of any high quality medical imaging system. Good design, proper calibration and maintenance of medical imaging systems may control and even eliminate artifacts.

Medical imaging systems often introduce distortion, another factor affecting image quality. Size distortion and shape distortion are illustrated in Fig. 3.8. Distortion can be very difficult to determine and correct. Developing methods for correcting distortion is very important for increasing image quality and improving diagnosis.

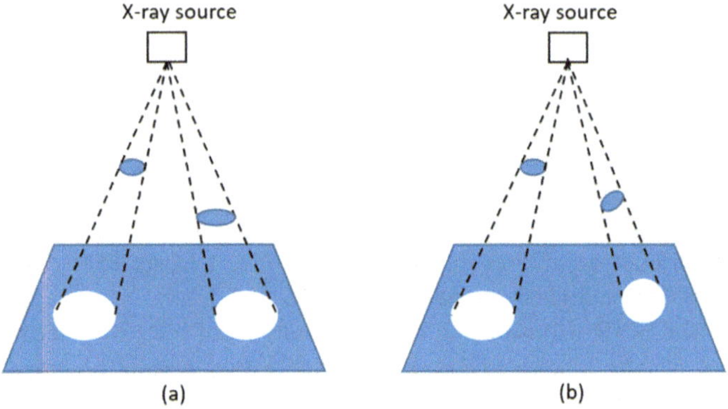

Fig. 3.8 **a** Size distortion in a radiographic imaging system due to magnification: although the sizes of the two dark objects are different, their projections are the same **b** Shape distortion in a radiographic imaging system due to x-ray beam divergence: although the two dark objects are the same, the shapes of their projections are different

3.3.7 Accuracy

In practice, quantitative accuracy and diagnostic accuracy are usually interesting.

Quantitative Accuracy: Sometimes, the numerical value of a given anatomic or functional feature within an image is interesting. In such situations, it is needed to know the error in the measurement. This error, or difference from the true value, arises from two sources: bias, which represents a systematic, reproducible difference from the truth, and imprecision, which represents a random, measurement-to-measurement variation. If the measurement is precise (i.e., reproducible), then systematic errors can be corrected through the use of a calibration standard that converts the measured value to the true value.

Diagnostic Accuracy: In a clinical setting, sensitivity and specificity are interesting. Sensitivity, also known as the true-positive fraction; this is the fraction of patients with disease whose test calls abnormal. Specificity, also known as the true-negative fraction; this is the fraction of patients without disease whose test calls normal. In practice, sensitivity and specificity are established in a group of patients through the use of a 2×2 contingency table, as shown in Fig. 3.9. Here, a and b are the number of diseased and normal patients whose test calls abnormal, whereas c and d are the number of diseased and normal patients whose test calls normal. In this case, sensitivity $= \frac{a}{a+c}$ and specificity $= \frac{b}{b+d}$. The diagnostic accuracy (DA) is the fraction of patients that are diagnosed correctly, and is given by

$$DA = \frac{a+d}{a+b+c+d}. \tag{3.46}$$

In practice, because of overlap in distribution of parameter values between normal and diseased patients, a threshold must be established to call a study "abnormal". A

Fig. 3.9 A contingency table

		Disease	
		abnormal	normal
Test	abnormal	a	b
	normal	c	d

lower threshold implies that more studies will be called abnormal, thus increasing sensitivity but decreasing specificity. A higher threshold implies that fewer studies will be called abnormal, thus increasing specificity but decreasing sensitivity. One way of graphically depicting this relation is via a receiver operating characteristic (ROC) curve. In practice, the threshold must be chosen as a balance between sensitivity and specificity. Two other parameters must be considered: Positive predictive value $\left(\mathrm{PPV} = \frac{a}{a+b}\right)$, which is the fraction of patients called abnormal who actually have the disease. Negative predictive value $\left(\mathrm{NPV} = \frac{d}{c+d}\right)$, which is the fraction of patients called normal who do not have the disease. And that both depend on prevalence (PR), which is given by

$$PR = \frac{a+c}{a+b+c+d}. \tag{3.47}$$

3.3.8 Examples

Now, the factors affecting image quality using projection radiography are described as an example. Assuming unity magnification and infinitesimal source size, a rectangular object, will cast a rectangular shadow on the detector with dimensions equal to the object dimensions. A 1D slice through the intensities on the detector will look like a rect function, as shown in Fig. 3.10. The local contrast of this object is given by

$$C = \frac{I_t - I_b}{I_b}. \tag{3.48}$$

Because the x-rays arrive in discrete quanta, there will be random fluctuations in the number of photons arriving in each small area of the detector, leading to noise. This effect is called quantum mottle, which is responsible for the imprecision of detector measurements of x-ray intensity.

The effect of the noise on image formation is quantified using the concept of SNR. The higher the SNR, the less evident the granularity in the image resulting from this quantum effect. The basic SNR in this scenario is given by

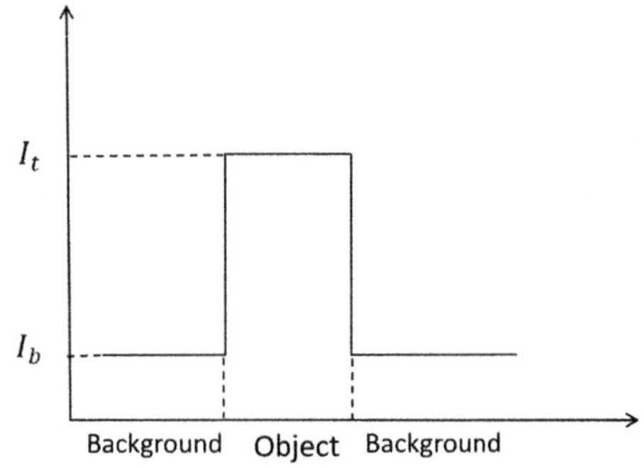

Fig. 3.10 Detector intensities from a rectangular object

$$\mathrm{SNR} = \frac{I_t - I_b}{\sigma_b} = \frac{\mathrm{CI}_b}{\sigma_b}. \tag{3.49}$$

In the background, the average number of photons per burst per area A can be denoted as N_b. Then the local SNR is given by

$$\mathrm{SNR} = C\sqrt{N_b}. \tag{3.50}$$

The above equation reveals a fundamental tradeoff in x-ray imaging. In order to improve the visibility of a particular structure in a radiograph, it is necessary to either increase the contrast of the structure or to increase the number of photons used in the visualization or analysis (or both).

The SNR can be expressed in more details by adding several additional concepts, which is given by

$$\mathrm{SNR} = C\sqrt{\phi A R t \eta}, \tag{3.51}$$

where Φ is the number of photons per Roentgen per cm^2, A is the unit area, R is the body's radiation exposure in Roentgens, t is the fraction of photons transmitted through the body, and η is the detector efficiency.

It is noted that Compton scattering degrades image quality. This produces two unwanted results: a decrease in image contrast and a decrease in SNR. Compton scatter adds a constant intensity I_S to both target and background intensity, yielding a new contrast of

$$C' = \frac{(I_t + I_s) - (I_b + I_s)}{I_b + I_s} = C\frac{I_b}{I_b + I_s} = \frac{C}{1 + \frac{I_s}{I_b}}. \tag{3.52}$$

The ratio I_S/I_b is called scatter-to-primary ratio; clearly, it should be kept as small as possible in order to preserve contrast. The derivation of SNR in the presence of Compton scattering is

$$SNR' = \frac{I_t - I_b}{\sigma_b} = C\frac{I_b}{\sigma_b} = C\frac{N_b}{\sqrt{N_b + N_s}} = \frac{C\sqrt{N_b}}{\sqrt{1 + N_s/N_b}}. \quad (3.53)$$

Here, the symbol N_S stands for the number of Compton scattered photons per burst per area A on the detector. The SNR with Compton scattering is related to the SNR without Compton scattering by

$$SNR' = SNR\frac{1}{\sqrt{1 + I_s/I_b}}. \quad (3.54)$$

3.4 Pre-processing Algorithms for Medical Imaging

Mammography is sufficiently specialized and widely used modality within projection radiography. It is used for the early detection of breast cancer either by direct detection of tumors in the images or by detection of microcalcifications. Now, more than half of all mammography systems are direct digital radiography systems. Digital systems have advanced processing algorithms for contrast enhancement and small-structure enhancement, as well as noise removal algorithms that improve the quality of images. In this section, several pre-processing algorithms for medical imaging using mammography are shown as follows.

3.4.1 Noise Removal Algorithms

Denoising plays a crucial role in the field of medical imaging in regard to the improvement of image quality.

Lee et al. [1] proposed **a fast non-local means (FNLM) denoising algorithm** which utilized neighborhood filtering and implemented for early breast cancer detection based on medical mammography. For comparison with conventional denoising methods, the Wiener filter and total variation (TV) denoising algorithm were used in this study. **Wiener filtering** was a linear algorithm based on statistical probability. This filtering approach transformed signals in the spatial domain into the frequency domain with the objective of minimizing the gap between the desired value and the actual value of a signal by filtering. But this approach required that the noise and image values should be stationary and also generated unexpected blur. The **TV denoising algorithm** was an iterative filtering approach which quantified the magnitude of the signal change among pixels in an image. This approach had the disadvantage that the temporal resolution may be reduced. Thus, a FNLM approach based on the combination of the summed square means (SSM) and fast Fourier transform (FFT) was proposed, as shown in formula (3.55).

$$NLM[u_{\text{true}}](x) = \frac{1}{C(x)} \int_{\Omega} e^{-\frac{\left(G_k^* |u_{\text{true}}(x+.) - u_{\text{true}}(y+.)|^2\right)(0)}{h^2}} u_{\text{true}}(y)dy \tag{3.55}$$

where $C(x)$ is the normalization constant,G_k is the Gaussian kernel, and h is the filtering parameter.

To evaluate the image performance, the temporal resolution, coefficient of variation (COV) and contrast to noise ratio (CNR) were examined. The COV was represented as an average value with a standard deviation. It was an evaluation element based on the method of leveling the relative distribution range of pixels, the acquisition of values by averaging the signal intensity among pixels in a specific range, and verification of relative noise distribution under the leveling condition designated as desirable. This implied that a lower value of COV means less noise. In the case of CNR, the contrast of the region of interest to the ambient noise could be compared with each other. That is, a higher CNR value implied a higher contrast. The COV and CNR were calculated as follows:

$$\text{CNR} = \frac{\left|S_{\text{target}} - S_{\text{background}}\right|}{\sqrt{\sigma_{\text{target}}^2 + \sigma_{\text{background}}^2}} \tag{3.56}$$

$$\text{COV} = \frac{\sigma_{\text{target}}}{S_{\text{target}}} \tag{3.57}$$

where S and σ are the mean and the standard deviation. By comparing with other denoising methods, the FNLM denoising algorithm showed remarkable performance with respect to image quality. For example, for quantitative evaluation of COV and CNR, FNLM denoising algorithm was approximately 2 times better.

Ramachandran et al. [2] proposed a new algorithm which used tree-based decision and tristate nonlinear values to eliminate high density outlier noise in mammogram images. The proposed algorithm was called as **Tristate filter** (TSF). The following briefs the proposed algorithm illustrated for salt and pepper noise removal. All the operation were performed in a fixed 2D Kernel of size 3 × 3.

Step 1: Initialize a 2D Kernel of size 3 × 3.
Step 2: The processed pixel p (a, b) is termed noisy or not using the following condition $0 < p\ (a, b) < 255$.
Step 3: If the processed pixel falls outside the specified condition then the pixel is termed as faulty (noisy) pixel.
Step 4: Arrange the pixel values of the current processing window in increasing order.
Step 5: Check the 4 neighbors of the p (a, b) for 0 or 255. If all the 4 neighbors are noisy then find the mean of the four neighbors.
Step 6: If any of the 4 neighbors are not noisy then the current processing window is checked for no noisy pixels. The number of no faulty pixels is stored in the variable called "count", based on the value of the count variable. There are 4 subconditions.

Case a: If the count is $<\ =2$ then corrupted pixel is replaced by unsymmetrical trimmed median.
Case b: If the count is between 3 and 5 (inclusive of both) then faulty pixel is replaced by Unsymmetrical trimmed modified Winsorized mean.
Case c: If the count is greater than or equal to 6 then the corrupted pixel is replaced by unsymmetrical Trimmed midpoint.
Case d: If entire pixels is either 0 (or all pixels are 255) then there are two sub conditions.
Case 1): If all the pixels are combination of 0 and 255 then the faulty pixel is replaced with unsymmetrical Trimmed global mean of the entire image.
Case 2): If the entire pixels are either 0 or 255 then the pixels are considered as part of the background vicinity and it is retained.
Step 7: Move to next pixel and repeat the steps from 1 to 6 for the remaining pixels in an image.

Padmavathy et al. [3] used **non-subsampled shearlet transform (NSST)** to reduce different noises which are commonly found in mammogram images. Speckle is a granular "noise" that inherently exists in and degrades the quality of the mammographic image. A model of the speckle noise is represented as

$$g(x, y) = f(x, y) * u(x, y) + n(x, y), \tag{3.58}$$

where $g(x, y)$ is the observed image, $f(x, y)$ is the noise free image, $u(x, y)$ is the multiplicative component, and $n(x, y)$ is the additive component of the speckle noise in spatial domain. NSST decomposed with Non Subsampled Laplacian Pyramid (NSLP) to obtain the high and low-frequency components of the mammography image. Then the shearlet coefficients and sub-bands were obtained using the directional filters. The NSST was formed by assigning the composite dilation of a 2D affine system as in (3.59).

$$A_{DS} = \left\{\psi_{j,k,m}(x) = |det D|^{j/2}\psi \times \left(S^k D^j x - m\right) : j, k \in \mathbb{Z}, m \in \mathbb{Z}^2\right\}, \tag{3.59}$$

where ψ is shearlet generating function, S is Shearlet matrix, D is anisotropic matrix, m is shift parameter, j is scale parameter, and k is directional parameter. Finally the shearlet transform function was formed as

$$\psi^{(0)}_{j,k,m}(x) = 2^{j(3/2)}\psi^{(1)}\left(S_0^k D_0^j x - m\right)\psi^{(1)}_{j,k,m}(x) = 2^{j(3/2)}\psi^{(0)}\left(S_1^k D_1^j x - m\right). \tag{3.60}$$

The following briefed the proposed algorithm illustrated for noise removal.
Step 1: The circular shift values is applied on the noisy image $s(x, y)$

$$s'(x, y) = circular\_shift(s(x, y), [x_{\text{shift}}, y_{\text{shift}}]). \tag{3.61}$$

Step 2: To obtain the NSST coefficient, the NSST algorithm performs decomposition of the image that has copied,

$$s^{\mathrm{NSST}}(x,y) = \mathrm{NSST}\big(s'(x,y)\big). \tag{3.62}$$

Step 3: Apply the thresholding scheme on every noisy NSST Coefficients $\big(s_{\gamma}^{\mathrm{NSST}}(x,y)\big)$ to obtain the threshold coefficients

$$\hat{s}_{\gamma}^{\mathrm{NSST}}(x,y) = \Theta_{thr}\big(s_{\gamma}^{\mathrm{NSST}}(x,y)\big) = \begin{cases} s_{\gamma}^{\mathrm{NSST}}(x,y), & \big|s_{\gamma}^{\mathrm{NSST}}(x,y)\big| \geq \beta\sigma\sigma_{\gamma} \\ 0, & \text{otherwise} \end{cases}, \tag{3.63}$$

where σ is the standard deviation of the boisterous image and σ_{γ} is the standard deviation of the loud sub-band at each scale decayed utilizing the NSST, as shown in formula (3.64).

$$\sigma_{\gamma} = \frac{1}{L_{\gamma}}\sqrt{\sum_{x=1}^{L_{\gamma}}\sum_{y=1}^{L_{\gamma}} s_{\gamma}^{\mathrm{NSST}}(x,y) s_{\gamma}^{\mathrm{NSST}^{*}}(x,y)}, \tag{3.64}$$

where $s_{\gamma}^{\mathrm{NSST}*}(x,y)$ is the complex conjugate of $s_{\gamma}^{\mathrm{NSST}}(x,y)$ and L_{γ} is a length of the sub-band. The scale dependent parameter β is computed by

$$\beta = \sqrt{\log\big(L_{\gamma}\big)}. \tag{3.65}$$

Step 4: To reconstruct the denoised image, inversion of decomposition is used,

$$\hat{s}'(x,y) = NSST^{-1}\big(\hat{s}_{\gamma}^{NSST}(x,y)\big). \tag{3.66}$$

Step 5: Subsequently taking the NSST − 1, playing out the opposite movement and coming about denoised image which is moved back to the original position, the approximated image follows as:

$$\hat{s}(x,y) = circular\_shift\big(\hat{s}'(x,y), \big[-x_{shift}, -y\_shift\big]\big). \tag{3.67}$$

The experimental results showed that the proposed algorithms can preserve the edges and textures very well while weakening the noise.

Guo et al. [4] proposed an adaptive weighted median filter image denoising method based on hybrid genetic algorithm to solve the problem that the traditional weighted median filter has low contrast and fuzzy boundary. The weighted denoising parameters can adaptively change according to the detailed information of lung lobes and ground-glass lesions, and it can adaptively match the cross and mutation probability of genetic combined with the steady-state regional population density, so as to obtain

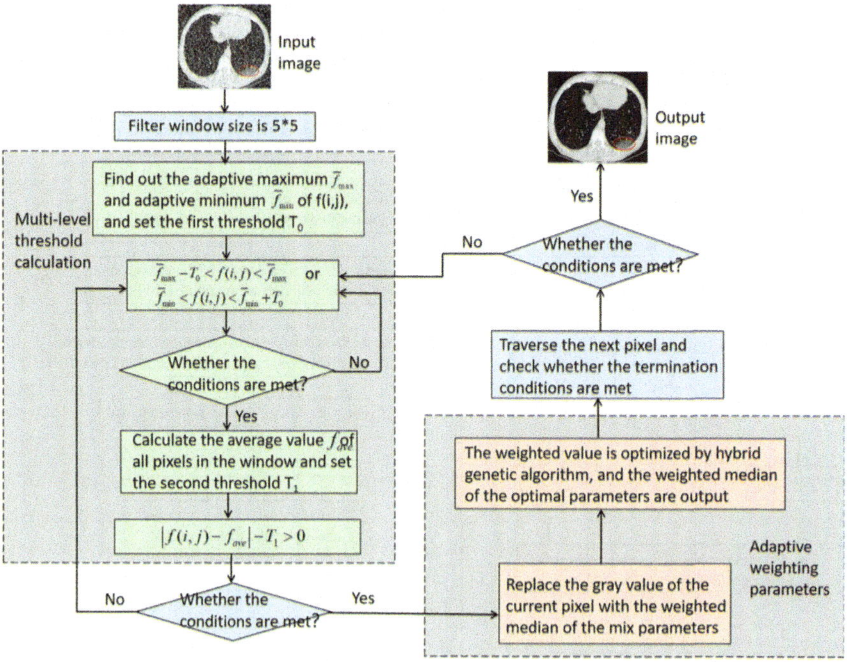

Fig. 3.11 Flow chart of median filtering based on adaptive threshold and optimized weighting parameters [5]

a more accurate COVID-19 denoised image with relatively few iterations. Figure 3.11 shows the flow chart of median filtering based on adaptive threshold and optimized weighting parameters.

Wang et al. [5] proposed a denoising method based on wavelet transform combined with improved particle swam optimization (PSO) to solve the problem that asymptomatic COVID-19 CT image often have small flake ground-glass shadow in the early lesions, and the density is low, which is easily confused with noise. Figure 3.12 shows the flow chart of wavelet transform combined with improved PSO. Aiming at the problems of low contrast and fuzzy boundary in the traditional wavelet transform, the threshold function based on the optimization of parameters combined with the improved PSO is proposed, so that the parameters of wavelet threshold function can change adaptively according to the lung lobe and ground-glass lesions with fewer iterations. The simulation results show that the paper method is significantly better than other algorithms in peak signal-to-noise ratio (PSNR), signal-to-noise ratio (SNR) and mean absolute error (MSE).

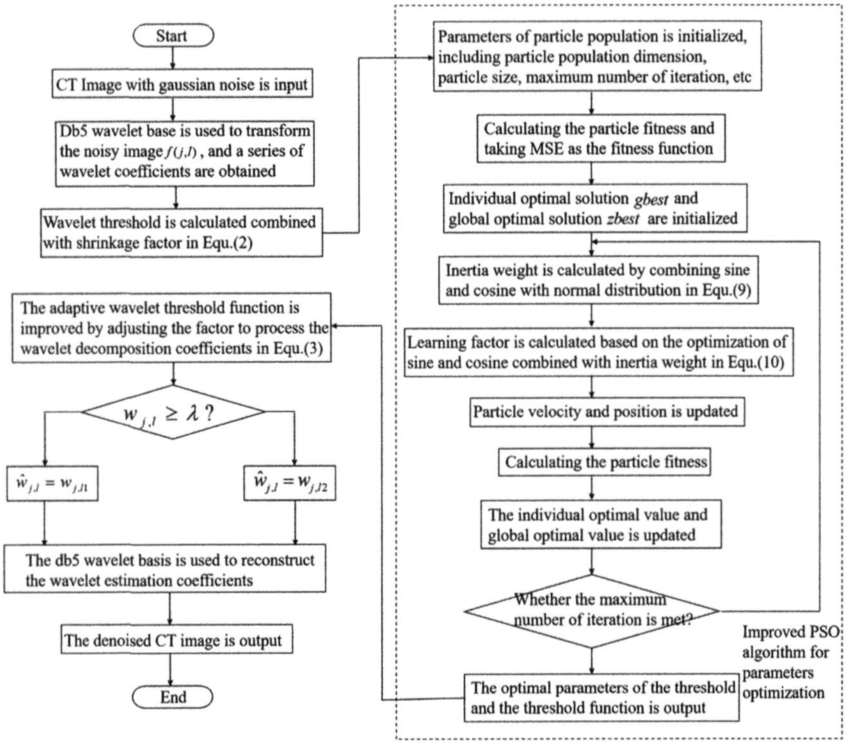

Fig. 3.12 Flow chart of wavelet transform combined with improved PSO [5]

3.4.2 Contrast Enhancement Algorithms

Medical image enhancement methods are mainly divided into two categories, contrast enhancement and small-structure enhancement. Contrast enhancement can enhance the differences between image levels, which is beneficial to clinicians' diagnosis and subsequent image processing. Algorithms for contrast enhancement in mammography can be divided into fuzzy enhancement, multi-scale geometric enhancement and so on according to different principle characteristics.

Sahba et al. [6] presented **a fuzzy operator** for contrast enhancement of mammography images. Its main idea consisted of three stages: fuzzification; a modification function application; and defuzzification. Therefore the algorithm can be summarized as follows:

Step 1: Calculate the image histogram.

Step 2: Initialize the membership values $\mu(g)$

$$\mu(g_{\text{mn}}) = \exp\left[-(g_{\text{Max}} - g_{\text{mn}})^2/2f_h^2\right], \tag{3.68}$$

where f_h and g_{Max} are a single fuzzifier and the maximum gray level presented in the image.

Step 3: Calculate the fuzziness γ

$$\gamma = \frac{4}{\text{MN}} \sum_{g=0}^{L-1} h(g)\mu_\lambda^*[1 - \mu_\lambda^*] \tag{3.69}$$

$$\mu_\lambda^*(g) = \frac{\mu(g)(1+\lambda)}{1+\lambda\mu(g)}, \tag{3.70}$$

where $h(g)$ is the frequency of g in the image.

Step 4: Find $f_{h_{\text{optimal}}}$ and λ_{optimal} to yield function γ

$$f_{h_{\text{optimal}}} = \left[\frac{\sum_{m=1}^{M} \sum_{n=1}^{N} (g_{\text{Max}} - g_{\text{mn}})^4}{\sum_{m=1}^{M} \sum_{n=1}^{N} (g_{\text{Max}} - g_{\text{mn}})^2} \right]^{0.5}. \tag{3.71}$$

$$\frac{\partial \gamma}{\partial \lambda}|_{\lambda=\lambda_{\text{optimal}}} = 0 \tag{3.72}$$

Step 5: Calculate the new membership values $\mu_{\text{new}}^*(g)\mu_{\text{new}}^*(g)$

$$\mu_{\text{new}}^*(g) = \frac{\mu(g)\left(1 + \lambda_{\text{optimal}}\right)}{1 + \lambda_{\text{optimal}}\mu(g)}. \tag{3.73}$$

Step 6: Generate the new gray level g' using the new membership values

$$g' = g_{\text{Max}} - \left\{-2\ln\left[\mu_{\text{new}}^*(g)\right] f_{h_{\text{optimal}}}^2\right\}^{1/2}. \tag{3.74}$$

The experimental results showed that this method can enhance the region of interest in mammography images that is useful for breast cancer diagnosis.

Wu et al. [7] proposed a new algorithm for feature and contrast enhancement of mammographic images **based on multi-scale transform and mathematical morphology**. To begin with, the original image was decomposed by the Laplacian Gaussian pyramid to obtain low-frequency sub-bands and different scales of the high-frequency sub-bands. For the low-pass filtered sub-band images, they applied the mathematical morphological operations, which combined opening operation with closing operation. And they adapted contrast limited adaptive histogram equalization (CLAHE) to enhance the high-frequency sub-bands coefficients. Finally, they reconstructed an image, whose size was same as the original image. Using the low-frequency coefficients adjusted contrast and the processed high-frequency sub-bands by the CLAHE to extract the enhanced images because the Laplacian Gaussian pyramid is of the property of reversal. The global gain operation was adopted to adjust the contrast of reconstructed image in order to make the enhanced image

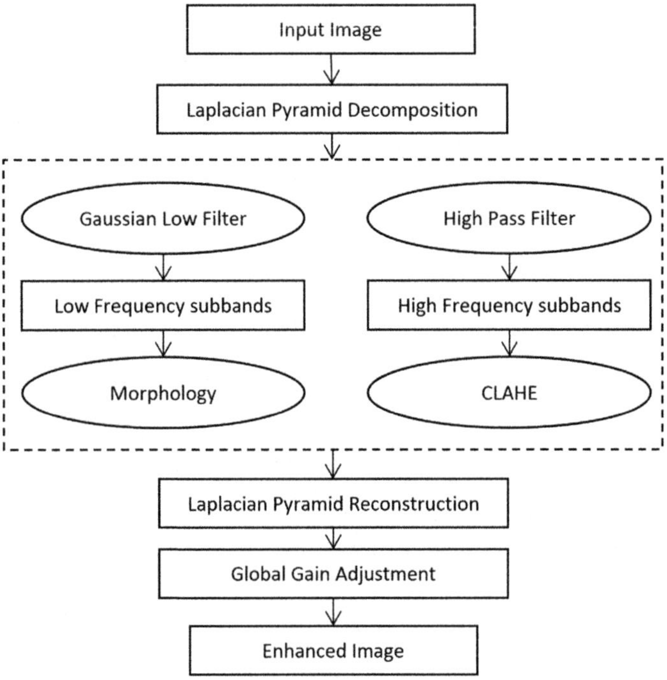

Fig. 3.13 The flowchart of the proposed algorithm

more natural and smoother. The flowchart of the proposed algorithm is shown in Fig. 3.13.

The Laplacian Gaussian Pyramid Transform: The Laplacian Gaussian pyramid has been used to analyze images at multi-scale for a broad range of application. The flow diagram of the Laplacian Gaussian pyramid for the decomposition and reconstruction processes of image is shown as Fig. 3.14. The original image is filtered by the Gaussian low-pass and subsampled to produce g_1. The image g_1 is next interpolated by convolution operation to reproduce the original array size, and pixelwise subtracted from the original image to produce b_0. This sub-band image b_0 is the finest level of the Laplacian Gaussian pyramid. The decimated low-pass image g_1 is further Gaussian low-pass filtered and subsampled producing g_2, and this is interpolated by convolution operation and subtracted from the g_1, resulting in the second pyramid layer b_1. All subsequent layers of the Laplacian Gaussian pyramid b_k are computed by repeating these operations to the subsampled Gaussian low-pass images g_k from the previous iteration, until the setting pyramid image b_{L-1} and the last pyramid image g_L are obtained. The flowchart of the reconstruction process is drawn in the right hand. The image g_L is interpolated to the array size of the next finer pyramid level b_{L-1}, and pixe is added to this. Interpolation, contrast enhancement and addition are repeated until the reconstructed image at the original resolution level is obtained.

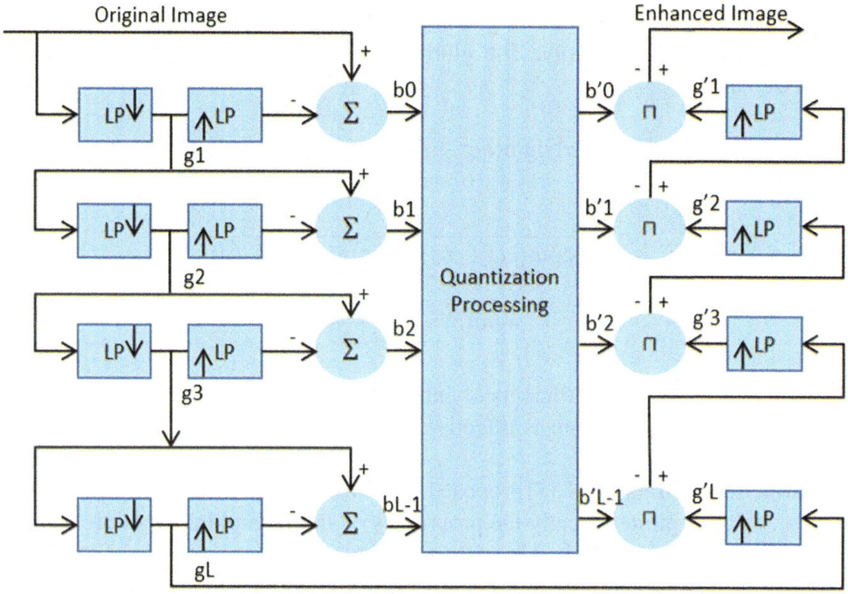

Fig. 3.14 The flow diagram of the Laplacian Gaussian pyramid for the decomposition and reconstruction processes of image

Mathematical Morphology: The morphological Dilation and Erosion operation applied to process the different sub-band images, which can enhance the contrast of image. In order to enhance the local contrast of the mammograms, the processing procedure is adding original image to the top-hat (*TH*) transformed image, and subtracting the bottom-hat (*BH*) image. The calculate formula (3.75) is given as follows:

$$
\begin{aligned}
C &= I + TH - BH \\
TH &= I - (I \circ SE) \\
BH &= (I \cdot SE) - I \\
I \circ SE &= (I \otimes SE) \otimes SE \\
I \cdot SE &= (I \oplus SE) \otimes SE \\
(I \otimes SE)(m, n) &= \min\{I(m - i, n + j) - SE(i, j)\}
\end{aligned}
$$

$$
(I \oplus SE)(m, n) = \max\{I(m - i, n - j) + SE(i, j)\}, \tag{3.75}
$$

where $SE(i, j)$ is a structural element.

Contrast Limited Adaptive Histogram Equalization: As described above, the limited function is defined to limit the gray level probability density, and the exceed histogram is adjusted to restrict noise.

Global Gain Adjustment: A global gain adjustment technique is presented to enhance all pixels uniformly. The global gain adjustment function $f(z)$ can be expressed as:

$$f(z) = a\big[\text{sigm}(c(z - b)) - \text{sigm}(-c(z + b))\big] \tag{3.76}$$

$$a = \frac{1}{\text{sigm}(c(1 - b)) - \text{sigm}(-c(z + b))} \tag{3.77}$$

$$\text{sigm}(z) = \frac{1}{1 + e^{-z}}, \tag{3.78}$$

where b and c are rate coefficients of enhancement. The experimental results show that the presented algorithm is effective for feature and contrast enhancement of mammogram.

Furthermore, Malali et al. [8] proposed a contrast enhancement model for mammograms, which exploited locally the proprieties of **the sigmoidal function** based on the **multi-objective Genetic Algorithm** for improving the contrast of lesions. The idea behind the proposed method was to minimize the impact of the low contrast on the perception of breast abnormality using either human or machine vision. To resolve this challenge, the image was subdivided into several non-overlapping blocks; within each block, there was a lower and an upper gray-level range. A nonlinear sigmoidal function was used to reduce the lower range of low gray-levels and the higher range of higher gray-levels; at the same time, the s-curve allowed to increase the gap between the lower and higher ranges. This difference in optical densities allowed improvement of contrast and sharpening the limiting edges. The local transformation function is below:

$$s = \frac{1}{1 + B^{\frac{-(r-\alpha)}{\beta}}}, \tag{3.79}$$

where r and s are the normalized gray levels of the target and resultant images normalized in the range of [0, 1]. α and β are respectively the center and width of sigmoid function. The modified local transformation function now required optimal tuning of its parameters so as to make the function adaptive to different natures of mammograms. The multi-objective genetic algorithm has been applied for optimal tuning of parameters of modified s-curve transformation. The Eq. (3.80) below is developed for managing the single objective optimization.

$$F = \omega_1 \text{EC}(I_{\text{out}}) + \omega_2 \text{AMBE}_n(I_{\text{in}}, I_{\text{out}}), \tag{3.80}$$

where ω_1 and ω_2 are nonzero weight factors, with $\omega_1 + \omega_2 = 1$, I_{in} and I_{out} are respectively the input and the output mammogram image(s), EC and AMBE_n are the measures of Image Quality Assessment (IQA).

3.4.3 Small-Structure Enhancement Algorithms

Small-structure enhancement can highlight some lesion structures and details, which is also beneficial to clinicians' diagnosis and subsequent image processing. According to different principles and characteristics, the enhancement methods of small structures in medical images can be divided into sharpening enhancement, rough set and fuzzy set enhancement, multi-scale geometric enhancement and other methods based on differential operators [9].

Sharpening enhancement is mainly to enhance the clarity of image edges and texture details. Since sharpening enhancement is sensitive to noise, it inevitably amplifies the noise while enhancing the structural details. Many scholars have made improvements to this, such as multi-scale anti-noise and anti-sharpening mask enhancement combined with non-subsampled contourlet transform (NSCT) [10]. Liu et al. proposed a medical image enhancement method using NSCT combined unsharp mask. The steps of the proposed algorithm can be summarized as follows:

Step 1: Decompose the input medical image using **NSCT**, obtaining a low-frequency sub-band and several high-frequency sub-bands. NSCT consists of two filter banks, the nonsubsampled pyramid filter bank (NSPFB) and the nonsubsampled directional filter bank (NSDFB). The NSPFB provides nonsubsampled multi-scale decomposition and captures the point discontinuities. The two-stage decomposition structure of NSPFB is shown in Fig. 3.15. The filters for subsequent stages are acquired by up-sampling the filters of the previous stage. This gives the multi-scale property without the need for additional filter design. First-stage low-pass and band-pass filters are denoted as $H_0(Z)$ and $H_1(Z)$, second-stage low-pass and band-pass filters are $H_0(Z^2)$ and $H_1(Z^2)$. The NSDFB provides nonsubsampled directional decomposition and links point discontinuities into linear structures. The l stage NSDFB produces 2^l directional sub-bands.

Step 2: Adopt contrast stretching using the equation to enhance contrast of the low-frequency sub-band. First, compute the minimum and the maximum of grayscale value, and then range the gray level from $[x_{\min}, x_{\max}]$ to [0, 255]. Each pixel x is modified using the linear mapping function:

$$f(x) = 255(x - x_{\min})/(x_{\max} - x_{\min}). \tag{3.81}$$

Step 3: For the high-frequency sub-bands, suppress image noise using **the adaptive thresholding method**. Adaptive thresholding T is calculates as follows:

$$T = \lambda T_B. \tag{3.82}$$

The weighted factors λ in different directions are computed by the Eq. (3.83):

$$\lambda = \frac{S_l}{S_{l,k}} \tag{3.83}$$

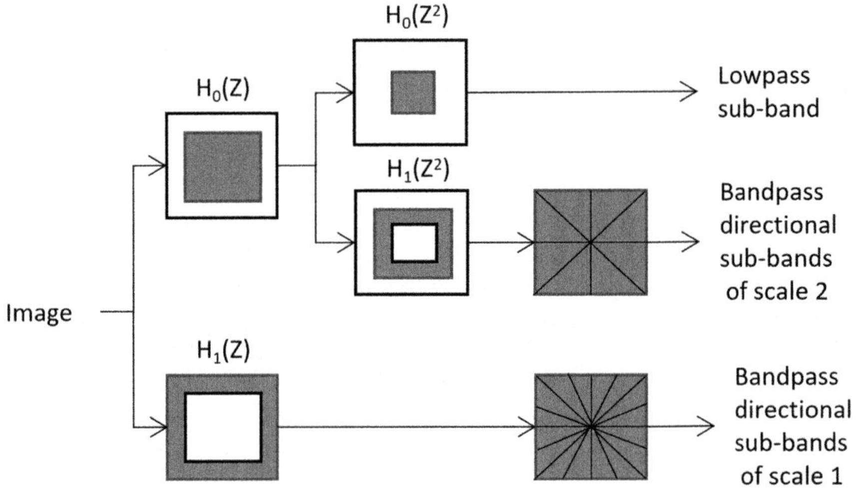

Fig. 3.15 The two-stage decomposition structure of NSPFB

The average coefficient S_l is:

$$S_l = \frac{\sum_{k=1}^{2^l} S_{l,k}}{2^l} \tag{3.84}$$

$$S_{l,k} = \frac{1}{m \times n} \sum_{i=1}^{m} \sum_{j=1}^{n} x_{i,j}(l,k) \tag{3.85}$$

k denotes the number of decomposition direction in the lst level.

The Bayes Shrink threshold T_B is computed as:

$$T_B = c \frac{\sigma^2}{\sigma_x^2} \tag{3.86}$$

σ^2 is the noise variance, σ_x^2 is the signal variance, as shown in formula (3.87) and (3.88).

$$\sigma = \frac{\text{median}\left|x_{i,j}(l,k)\right|}{0.6745} \tag{3.87}$$

$$\sigma_x = \sqrt{\max\left(\frac{1}{mn} \sum_{i=1}^{m} \sum_{j=1}^{n} x_{i,j}^2(l,k) - \sigma^2, 0\right)}. \tag{3.88}$$

Then adopt the threshold T of previous choice to suppress noise, as shown in formula (3.89).

$$x'_{i,j} = \begin{cases} x_{i,j}, x_{i,j} > T \\ 0, x_{i,j} < T \end{cases}. \quad (3.89)$$

Step 4: Reconstruct all coefficients using **the inverse transformation of NSCT.**

Step 5: Obtain the final enhanced image using **the unsharp masking method.** The unsharp masking method is accomplished by subtracting the Laplace filtering component from the original image using the following Eq. (3.90):

$$g(x, y) = f(x, y) + K \times \left(f(x, y) - f'(x, y)\right), \quad (3.90)$$

where $f'(x, y)$ represents artificial vague image.

Another kind of small-structure enhancement method is the enhancement method based on fuzzy mathematics and rough set theory. **Rough set-based enhancement** divides the image into different parts according to the unique attributes of the medical image, and enhances and highlights the texture details of the small region of interest [11]. In the work of Ashish Phophalia et al., a rough set theory (RST)-based approach was used to obtain pixel level rough edge map (REM) and rough class labels (RCL). REM strongly controls the effect of bilateral filter on edge and non-edge pixels whereas the RCL keeps track of the homogeneity within object and heterogeneity on the edges. The performance of existing bilateral filter is boosted up by prior information derived by REM and RCL. **The enhancement based on the fuzzy set** transforms the image into the fuzzy domain, performs appropriate enhancement processing on the image in the fuzzy domain, and then inversely transforms the image from the fuzzy domain to the spatial domain according to the membership function to obtain the enhanced image [12]. In the work of Tamalika Chaira, to have better information on uncertainty on the membership function, **Type II fuzzy set** was considered. Hamacher T co norm was used as an aggregation operator to form a new membership function using the upper and lower membership function of Type II fuzzy set. The image is initially fuzzified using the formula (3.91):

$$\mu'\left(g_{ij}\right) = \frac{g - g_{\min}}{g_{\max} - g_{\min}}. \quad (3.91)$$

The upper and lower ranges of Type II fuzzy membership function are calculated using Eq. (3.92) and (3.93) with $\alpha = 0.8$.

$$\mu^{\text{upper}} = [\mu(x)]^{\alpha} \quad (3.92)$$

$$\mu^{\text{lower}} = [\mu(x)]^{1/\alpha}. \quad (3.93)$$

Next, a membership function is computed that considers both the upper and lower membership functions using the Hamacher T co norm, as shown in formula (3.94).

$$\mu^{enh}(g_{ij}) = \frac{\mu^{\text{upper}} + \mu^{\text{lower}} + (\lambda - 2)\mu^{\text{upper}}\mu^{\text{lower}}}{1 - (1 - \lambda)\mu^{\text{upper}}\mu^{\text{lower}}} \tag{3.94}$$

and λ is the average of the image. This method reduces the amount of computation, shortens the image processing time and effectively enhances the image.

In addition, there are two types of methods based on **multi-scale geometric enhancement methods** such as wavelet transform and **enhancement methods based on differential operators**. Wavelet transform can effectively decompose an image into low-frequency parts containing approximate information and high-frequency parts containing texture details, and perform multi-scale analysis of images in both spatial and frequency domains [13]. The general idea of **wavelet transform image enhancement** is to selectively adjust the wavelet decomposition coefficient by constructing a linear or nonlinear transform function reasonably to highlight the small structures in the enhanced image. By using the wavelet transform and Haar transform, a novel image enhancement approach was proposed in the work of Anamika Bhardwaj et al. The specific steps are as follows:

Step 1: A medical image is decomposed with **Haar transform**.

Step 2: Then high-frequency subimages are decomposed with **wavelet transform**. The image decomposition is shown in the Fig. 3.16.

In order to obtain more image detail information, all high-frequency sub images are decomposed up to 3 level.

Step 3: The noise in the frequency field is reduced by **the soft-threshold method**. The threshold is computed by

$$T = \beta\sigma^2\sigma y, \tag{3.95}$$

where σ and σy are the standard deviation of the noise and the sub-band data of noisy image. β is the scale parameter, which depends upon the sub-band size and number of decomposition, as shown in formula (3.96).

$$\beta = \sqrt{\log(\text{Lk}/\text{J})} \tag{3.96}$$

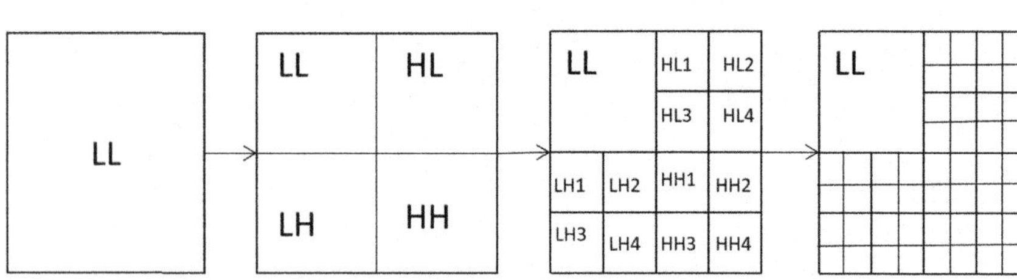

Fig. 3.16 The image decomposition with wavelet transform

Lk is length of sub-band, J is total number of decomposition.

Step 4: Then high-frequency coefficients are enhanced by different weight values in different sub images. Denoised high-frequency coefficient are **multiply by 1.5** (assign weight value) to get enhanced coefficient.

Step 5: Then the enhanced image is obtained through **the inverse Haar transform**.

Step 6: Lastly, the image's contrast is adjust by **nonlinear contrast enhancement approaches**. Nonlinear contrast enhancement often involves histogram equalization through the use of an algorithm, such as Histogram equalization method, Adaptive histogram equalization method, Homomorphic Filter method and Unsharp Mask.

The method based on the differential operators can calculate the intensity and direction or structure tensor of the grayscale change of the image local neighborhood, which is equivalent to adding directional information to the structure of a two-dimensional image, and it can effectively enhance the structure in the image [14]. Rodrigo Moreno et al. proposed a **filtered structure tensor (FST)** based on gradient enhancement of tubular structures in medical images. Let u(x, y) be a two-dimensional image function, and its **structure tensor** can be composed of the first-order partial derivatives of its pixels:

$$\begin{aligned} \mathrm{ST} &= \nabla u(x, y) \otimes \nabla u(x, y) = \nabla u(x, y) \cdot \nabla u^T(x, y) \\ &= \begin{bmatrix} \left(\frac{\partial u}{\partial x}\right)^2 & \frac{\partial u}{\partial x} \cdot \frac{\partial u}{\partial y} \\ \frac{\partial u}{\partial y} \cdot \frac{\partial u}{\partial x} & \left(\frac{\partial u}{\partial y}\right)^2 \end{bmatrix} \\ &= \begin{bmatrix} e_1 \; e_2 \end{bmatrix} \cdot \begin{bmatrix} \lambda_1 & 0 \\ 0 & \lambda_2 \end{bmatrix} \cdot \begin{bmatrix} e_1^T \\ e_2^T \end{bmatrix}, \end{aligned} \tag{3.97}$$

where $\nabla u(x, y)$ represents the gradient vector of the image $u(x, y)$ and $\otimes$ represents the tensor product. The eigenvector e_1 and e_2 of the matrix represents the direction of signal change in the neighborhood, and its eigenvalues λ_1 and λ_2 represent the size information that changes along these directions, reflecting the characteristics of pixel changes in this field. According to the information of eigenvalues and eigenvectors, the local geometric structure of the image can be described to perform targeted enhancement on the region of interest in the image. They proposed to use $\widehat{\rightarrow}_r$ to filter out the gradients that are not likely part of the vessel. Thus, they propose the following structure tensor:

$$\mathrm{FST}\left(\overrightarrow{X}\right) = G * \nabla I' \nabla I'^T, \tag{3.98}$$

where G is a Gaussian kernel, "*" is the convolution operation, and I′ is the filtered gradient, which is computed as:

$$\nabla I' = H\left(t \nabla I^T \vec{r}\right) \nabla I, \tag{3.99}$$

where H is the Heaviside function, $\rightarrow_r = \rightarrow_{x'} - \rightarrow_x$ and t takes its value depending on the type of vessel of interest: $t = -1$ for bright and $t = 1$ for dark vessels. The main advantage of the proposed structure tensor is that it is less sensitive to biases generated by gradients from nearby structures.

3.5 Computed-Aided Diagnosis Algorithms for Medical Imaging

Several computed-aided diagnosis (CAD) algorithms for medical imaging using mammography are shown as an example. In reality, many CAD systems are used to aid physicians in the early diagnosis of breast tumors on mammograms. In addition, deep learning has a higher diagnostic accuracy for detecting breast cancer on mammograms. Therefore, several researches have established deep learning-based CAD for their efficiency and accuracy in predicting the growth of cancer cells utilizing medical imaging modalities. This section describes the main categories of existing deep learning-based breast cancer detection, lesion classification and image segmentation methods, including artificial neural networks, deep belief networks, convolutional neural networks, extreme learning machines and generative adversarial networks [15].

3.5.1 Artificial Neural Network (ANN)

An ANN is a mathematical model based on the structure and capabilities of a biological neural networks, which plays an essential role in the diagnosis of breast cancer. The basic architecture of an ANN with multiple hidden layers is given in Fig. 3.17.

Rouhi et al. [16] presented two automated methods with limited images to classify benign and malignant cancers in mammograms. In the first proposed method, segmentation is done using an automated **region growing** whose threshold

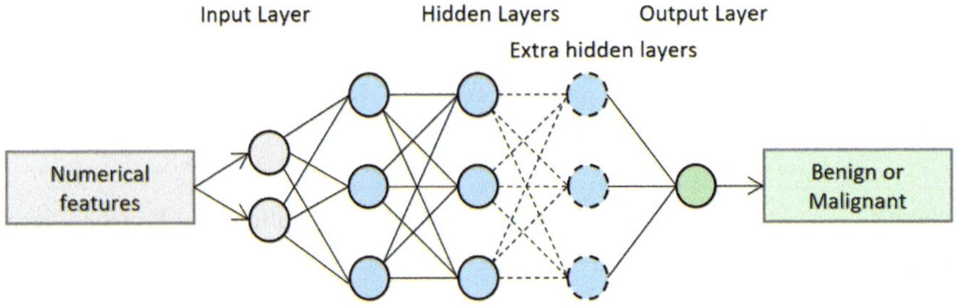

Fig. 3.17 A sample illustration of ANN with multiple hidden layers for breast cancer diagnosis

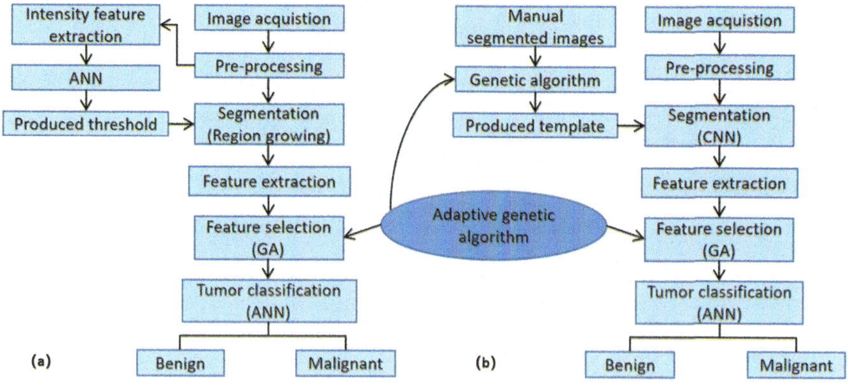

Fig. 3.18 **a** The first proposed automated technique based on region growing segmentation **b** The second proposed automated technique based on cellular neural network segmentation

is obtained by a trained ANN. In the second proposed method, segmentation is performed by a **cellular neural network** (CNN) whose parameters are determined by a genetic algorithm (GA). Intensity, textural and shape features are extracted from segmented tumors. GA is used to select appropriate features from the set of extracted features. In the next stage, ANNs are used to classify the mammograms as benign or malignant. The general trend of the proposed automatic techniques is introduced in Fig. 3.18. In the future work, we think that adaptive genetic algorithm can be used to determine the parameters of CNN and select appropriate features.

3.5.2 Deep Belief Network (DBN)

The DBN is unsupervised graphical model, which is essentially generative in nature. The DBN is a multi-layer belief network, where each layer is a restricted Boltzmann machine (RBM), and they are stacked with each other to form the DBN. The initial stage in training DBN is to learn a set of features from visible units using the contrastive divergence (CD) method. Then, the activations of previously trained features are treated as visible units, and, in a second hidden layer, the DBN learns more robust features from the previously acquired visible units. The architecture of DBN is presented in Fig. 3.19.

Al-antari et al. [17] proposed a CAD system for breast cancer diagnosis via DBN that automatically detected breast mass regions and recognized them as normal, benign, or malignant. The schematic diagram of the DBN-based CAD system is shown in Fig. 3.20, which involves **automatic mass detection**, region of interest **(ROI) extraction techniques, feature extraction and DBN classifier modules**. The presented system is slightly different in the use of ROIs and involves two techniques, Mass ROIs and Whole Mass ROIs. We think that we could use the combination of principal component analysis and linear discriminant analysis to extract features.

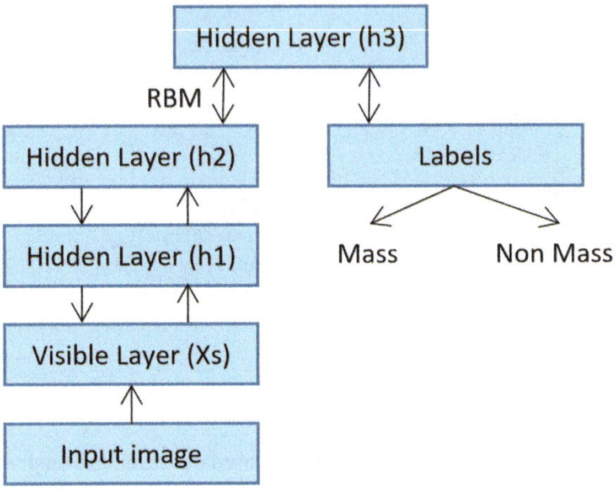

Fig. 3.19 An illustration of the DBN model for breast cancer diagnosis

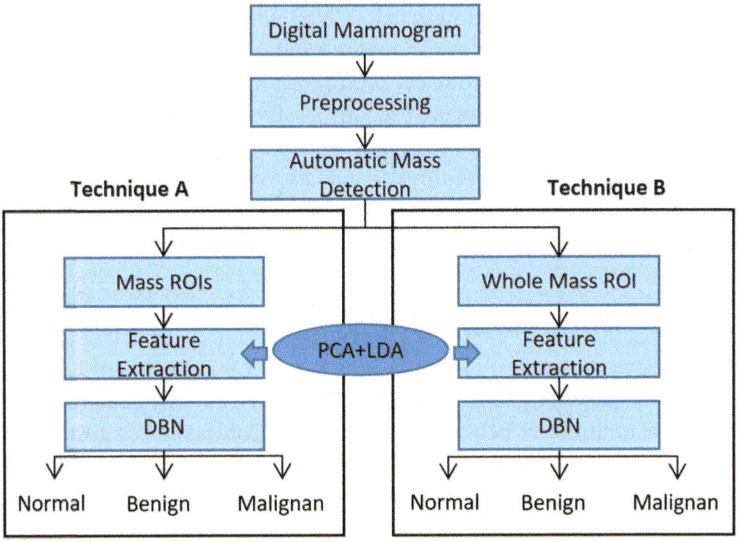

Fig. 3.20 The schematic diagram of the DBN-based CAD system processes

Automatic mass detection: One of the important steps in CAD for breast cancer classification is to detect specific masses or suspicious regions on mammograms. In this work, the automatic mass detection algorithm is shown in Fig. 3.21. They computed the threshold value L_{thr} by aggregating all gray level intensities inside the breast tissues and dividing them by the total number of nonzero pixels (L), which is known as the gray scale intensity of the local background, as follows:

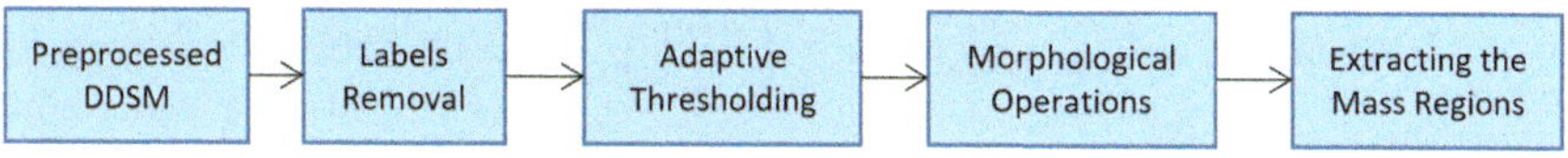

Fig. 3.21 The automatic mass detection algorithm

$$L_{thr} = \frac{\sum_{i,j \in I} I(i,j)}{L}. \tag{3.100}$$

Then, they applied this threshold to the breast image, converting the threshold image to the binary image in order to apply morphological operations. Consecutive binary morphological operations were applied to determine the proper shape and size of the mass. These operations were accomplished using three steps. First, they utilized a fill operation to complete the whole expected suspicious region. Second, erosion with a structuring element of disk type was applied. Finally, they removed the remaining disconnected small areas remaining around the mass after the erosion process.

DBN classifier modules: They utilized R and Q hidden nodes with first and second hidden layers. The training of DBN was achieved through two consecutive processes. First, a pre-training process for RBM was performed via unsupervised learning. Then, they utilized a supervised learning method to apply a back propagation algorithm with known labels of breast cancer features to adjust the weights and fine-tune the networks. In fact, there are following five consecutive steps to train RBM:

Step 1: All parameters of the network are initialized and set to zero.

Step 2: The logical state of the first hidden layer is computed as follows:

$$h_1 = \begin{cases} 1; f\left(B + v_1 w^T\right) > \varphi \\ 0; \text{otherwise} \end{cases}, \tag{3.101}$$

where $f(z) = 1/\left(1 + e^{-z}\right)$ is a sigmoid activation function, and φ is an activation threshold.

Step 3: The state of visible layer v_{recon} is reconstructed corresponding to the following formula (3.102):

$$v_{\text{recon}} = \begin{cases} 1; f(A + h_1 w) > \varphi \\ 0; \text{otherwise} \end{cases} \tag{3.102}$$

Step 4: Compute the state of hidden layer h_{recon} as follows:

$$h_{\text{recon}} = f\left(B + v_{\text{recon}} w^T\right). \tag{3.103}$$

Step 5: The difference of weight Δw is estimated to compute the current one as follows:

$$w_{k+1} = \Delta w + w_k,\ \Delta w = \left(\frac{h_1 v_1}{\eta}\right) - \left(\frac{h_{\text{recon}} v_{\text{recon}}}{\eta}\right), \tag{3.104}$$

where η is the batch size.

3.5.3 Convolutional Neural Network (CNN)

A CNN is made up of three layers: the convolution layer, the max-pooling layer and the output layer, which used to extract useful features from medical images and perform breast cancer classification. **De-novo CNNs** (CNNs trained from scratch) and **TL-based CNNs** (pre-trained CNNs) are mainly used in breast cancer classification. A basic workflow with CNN in breast cancer diagnosis is given in Fig. 3.22.

De-novo CNN is a CNN with few layers or multiple layers by training it from scratch. Ting et al. [18] presented the algorithm called convolutional neural network improvement for breast cancer classification (CNNI-BCC) to assist medical experts in breast cancer diagnosis in timely manner. The application of present algorithm can assist classification of mammographic medical images into benign patient, malignant patient and healthy patient without prior information of the presence of a cancerous lesion. Figure 3.23 shows the overall procedure of the CNNI-BCC method. It consists of three main steps: **feature wise pre-processing (FWP), CNN-based classification (CNNBS), interactive detection-based lesion locator (IDBLL)**. FWP is designed to shorten the CNN process time by pre-processing the input images beforehand. FWP is applied to divide the input image into smaller image patches. The images patches are rotated clockwise to 90°, 180°, 270° and 360°. Every rotated patch is flipped vertically. CNNI-BCC architecture is constructed from one input layer, two hidden layer and one output layer. The hidden layer has convolutional layer, rectified linear unit layer, pooling layer and fully connected layer. The MIAS dataset is divided into training set and testing set. Feature wise data augmentation is applied to increase the data pool to reduce the overfitting occurrence. The trained model is utilized during testing phase for classification status. The trained model is further

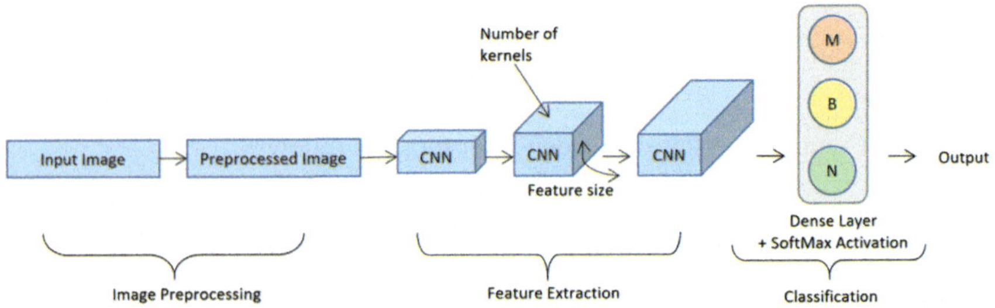

Fig. 3.22 An illustration of CNN-based model for breast cancer diagnosis

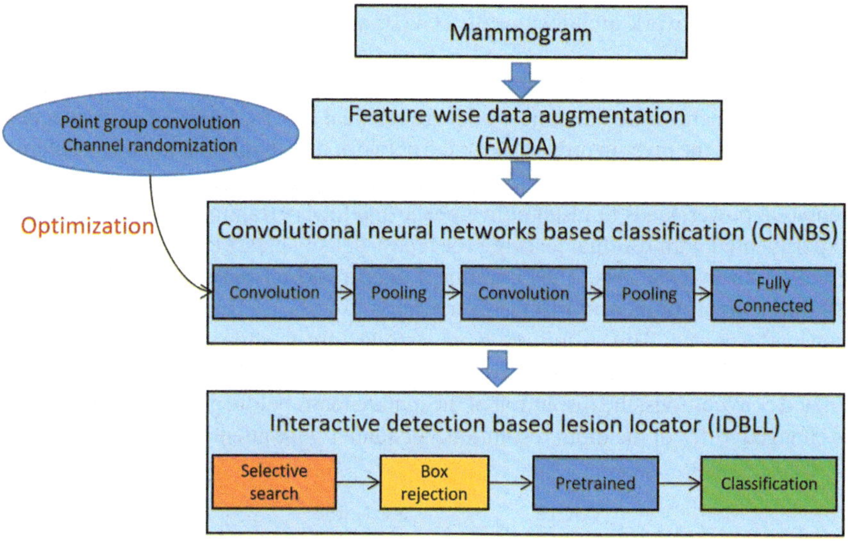

Fig. 3.23 The overall procedure of the CNNI-BCC method

implemented through IDBLL, which can detect object by using predicted bounding boxes. The features are resampled for each predicted bounding box, and classified through IDBLL. We could optimize the neural network in the algorithm by using methods such as point group convolution and channel randomization in the future work.

Transfer learning (TL) is an efficient approach for dealing with small datasets by allowing pre-trained networks to be fine-tuned and adjusted to solve problems from a particular domain or imaging modality. The weights of the model are pre-initialized when utilizing a pre-trained version, as opposed to being randomly initialized while training from scratch. The study proved that the classifier performed better on features extracted with a **TL-based CNN**. Chougrad et al. [19] developed a computer-aided diagnosis system based on pre-trained CNNs that aimed to help the radiologist classify mammography mass lesions. In this study, they used some state-of-art architectures, which were pre-trained on ImageNet, i.e., VGG16, ResNet50, Inception v3, for transfer learning from natural images to breast cancer images. Figure 3.24 gives the schema for the models setup using **transfer learning** while adopting a **fine-tuning strategy** for some of the last convolutional blocks. The three differently-colored dotted rectangular selections represent the different implementations of the models, i.e., in each implementation the selected layers in the rectangle are fine-tuned while the rest of the model's layers are frozen. They proposed to fine-tune the models to adjust the features of the last convolutional blocks and made them more data-specific; they fine-tuned the weights of the pre-trained networks using the new set of images by resuming the backpropagation on the unfrozen layers. In the future, we could optimize the network architecture of VGG16 and ResNet50 by regularization and step optimization.

Recently few studies utilized **residual learning** for breast cancer diagnosis. The main components of residual networks are residual blocks. It uses skip connections to leap across the layer in order to keep the network from experiencing the problem of a vanishing gradient. The addition of residual blocks in the network increases representation power, leads to faster convergence and lowers training errors. Li et al. [20] experimented with residual learning for breast-density classification using mammograms from two datasets. They combined **deep residual networks** with integrated **dilated convolutions and attention methods** to improve the network's classification performance. The overall network architecture is shown in Fig. 3.25, which is composed of the input, feature extraction and classification modules. By utilizing dilated convolutions, the resolution of the feature maps before global average pooling is changed to 1/8 of the input resolution. A channel-wise attention block was applied

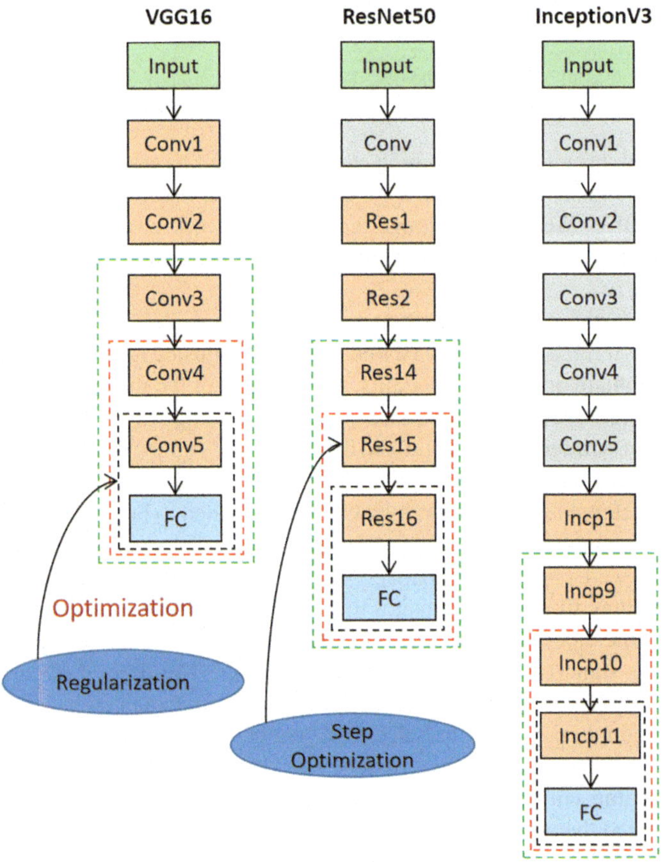

Fig. 3.24 The schema for the models setup using transfer learning

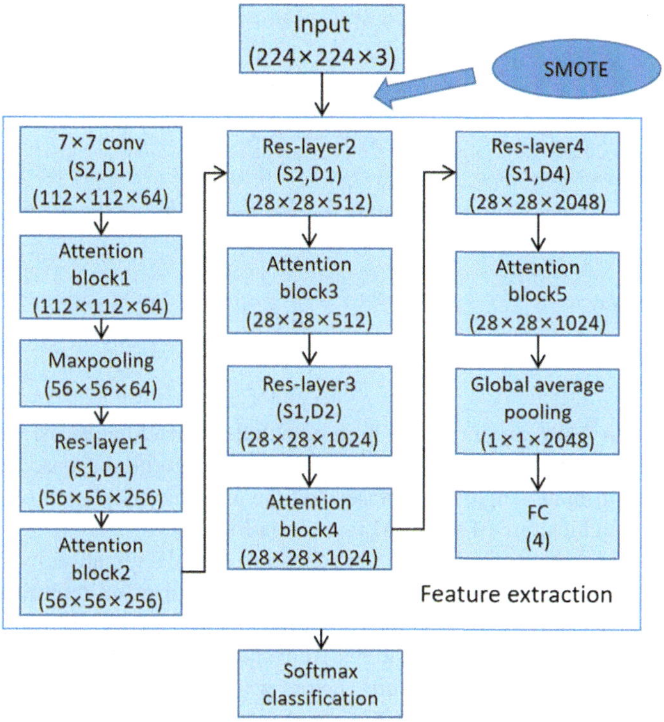

Fig. 3.25 The overall network architecture

to highlight the important feature maps in different layers. We will take a deeper look at the problem of data set imbalance, or we will use the SMOTE method to solve it.

For **a dilated convolution** with a dilation rate d, the operation can be represented as

$$(C_l * k)(p) = \sum_{s+d\cdot t=p} C_l(s)k(t) \tag{3.105}$$

where C_l refers to the feature map at layer l, and k refers to the filter with a dilation rate d. The receptive field of the element in the output feature map with regards to the input feature map is $ks + (ks + 1)(d - 1)$ with ks representing the kernel size. The **channel-wise attention block** in each layer adaptively learns a weight for each feature map in that layer to selectively utilize the extracted feature information. The output of the attention block is

$$Y_C = X_C + S \cdot X_C \tag{3.106}$$

where X_C is the input to the attention block and Y_C is the output of the block. S is the weight of each feature map calculated by

$$S = \sigma(W_2 * \delta(W_1 * Z + b_1) + b_2 \tag{3.107}$$

$$Z = \frac{1}{H \times W} \sum_{i=1}^{H} \sum_{j=1}^{W} (X_C), \tag{3.108}$$

where σ refers to the Sigmoid function. W_1, W_2, b_1 and b_2 are the weights and bias of the fully connected (FC) layers.

3.5.4 *Extreme Learning Machine (ELM)*

The ELM is an ANN variant with a high potential for handling breast cancer classification. It is a feed-forward neural network and the algorithm is based on random initialization of input weights and biases and the analytic calculation of the output weights. The architecture of the ELM is given in Fig. 3.26.

Muduli et al. [21] performed feature reduction and classification by **fusing the extreme learning machine and the moth flame optimization technique** (MFO-ELM) for breast cancer classification. The proposed model utilized lifting wavelet transform (LWT) to extract the features from the region of interest mammogram images. The dimension of the feature vectors was then reduced by using a fusion of principal component analysis (PCA) and linear discriminant analysis (LDA) methods. Finally, the classification was performed using an efficient optimized learning-based classifier MFO-ELM. The overview of the proposed model is defined

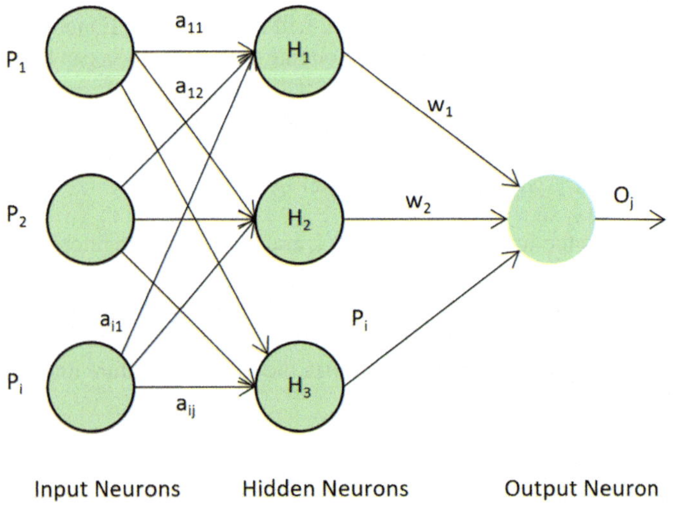

Fig. 3.26 A basic extreme learning machine architecture

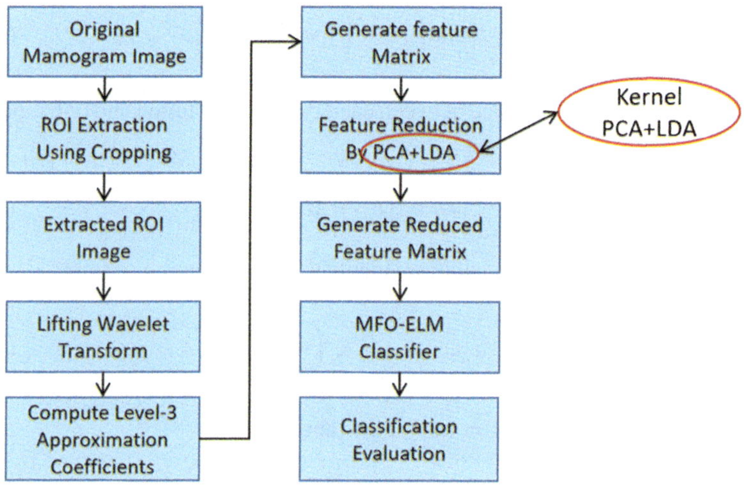

Fig. 3.27 The overview of the proposed model

in Fig. 3.27. In the future work, we consider using a fusion of kernel principal component analysis and LDA to reduce the dimension.

The MFO algorithm is used to select the hidden layer parameters like weights and bias values to maximize the performance of ELM. The main steps of the proposed MFO-ELM are as follows:

Step 1: Initialization: a random set of moths position called as candidate solutions with each position representing a neuron's hidden layer. Each candidate solution consists of a set of input weights and hidden biases with the given range [−1, 1], as shown in formula (3.109).

$$M_j = \left(W_{11}^h, W_{12}^h, W_{13}^h, \cdots, W_{1L}^h, \cdots, W_{21}^h, W_{22}^h, W_{23}^h, \cdots, W_{2L}^h, \cdots, W_{i1}^h, W_{i2}^h, W_{i3}^h, \cdots, W_{iL}^h, B_1, B_2, B_3, \cdots, B_L\right). \tag{3.109}$$

Step 2: Initialize current iteration $I = 1$, constant $b = 1$, the maximum iteration T.

Step 3: For each moth, the sum square error (SSE) $\mu(M_j)$ is calculated as follows:

$$\mu(M_j) = \sum_{j=1}^{N_{\text{val}}} \sum_{i=1}^{N_{\text{out}}} \left|O_{ij} - D_{ij}\right|. \tag{3.110}$$

Here N_{val} and N_{out} is the number of data points in the validation set and nodes in the output layer. O_{ij} and D_{ij} are called as actual output and expected output on node i with sample j.

Step 4: While $I < T$ then update the number of flames by

$$N_F = \text{round}\left(N - \left(I * \frac{N-1}{T}\right)\right). \quad (3.111)$$

Step 5: Calculate the distance between each candidate solution and corresponding flame by

$$D_i = \left|F_j - M_i\right|. \quad (3.112)$$

Step 6: For each candidate solution, identify the parameter a, r from

$$a = -1 + I \times \left(\frac{-1}{T}\right) \quad (3.113)$$

$$r = (a-1) \times \text{rand}() + 1 \quad (3.114)$$

and update the moth position using

$$S_p\left(M_i, F_j\right) = D_i e^{br} \cos(2\pi r) + F_j. \quad (3.115)$$

Step 7: Repeat step 3 to 6 up to the maximum number of iteration performed and to obtain the best optimal parameters for the proposed model.

3.5.5 *Generative Adversarial Network (GAN)*

Generative adversarial networks are deep-learning-based generative models. The GAN model framework consists of two submodels, i.e., the generator model and the discriminator model. The generator model produces new images from the features learned in the training data that resemble the original image. The discriminator model predicts whether the generated image is fake or real. As GANs do not require labeled data, they are particularly valuable for breast cancer classification. A GAN architecture is given in Fig. 3.28.

Singh et al. [22] used cGAN for breast tumor segmentation inside a mammogram's ROI. The proposed CAD system shown in Fig. 3.29 is divided into two stages: **breast tumor segmentation** and **shape classification**. The generative network learns to recognize the tumor area and to create the binary mask that outlines it. In turn, the adversarial network learns to distinguish between real (ground truth) and synthetic segmentations, thus enforcing the generative network to create binary masks as realistic as possible. Then, using a CNN-based shape discriminator, they classify the binary masks.

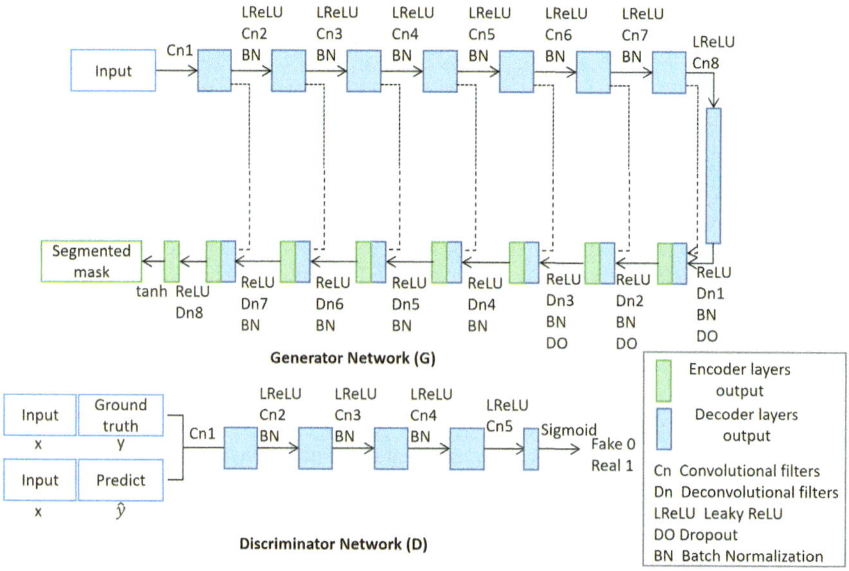

Fig. 3.28 A cGAN Architecture: generator G (top) and discriminator D (bottom) [15]

Fig. 3.29 The proposed CAD system

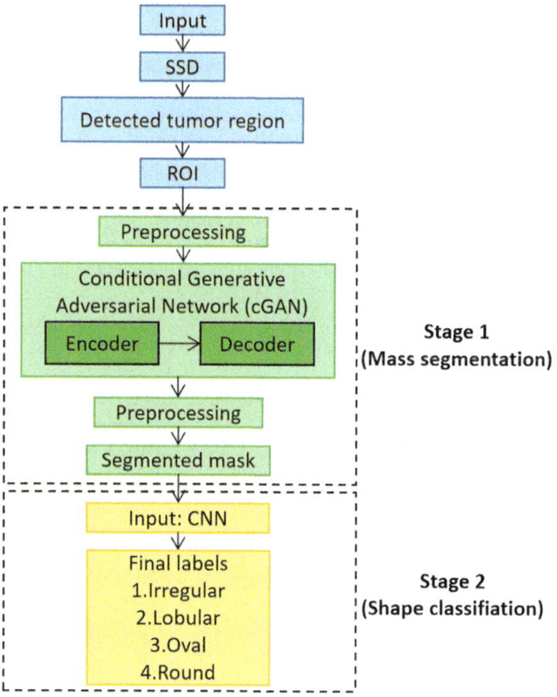

References

1. Lee S, Park SJ, Jeon JM, Lee MH, Ryu DY, Lee E, Kang SH, Lee Y. Noise removal in medical mammography images using fast non-local means denoising algorithm for early breast cancer detection: a phantom study[J]. Optik. 2019;180:569–75.
2. Ramachandran V, Kishorebabu V. A tri- state filter for the removal of salt and pepper noise in mammogram images[J]. J Med Syst. 2019;43:40.
3. Padmavathy TV, Vimalkumar MN, Nagarajan S, Badu GC, Parthasarathy P. Performance analysis of pre-cancerous mammographic image enhancement feature using non-subsampled shearlet transform[J]. Multimedia Tools Appl. 2021;80:26997–7012.
4. Guo S, Wang G, Han L, Song X, Yang W. COVID-19 CT image denoising algorithm based on adaptive threshold and optimized weighted median filter[J]. Biomed Signal Process Control. 2022;75: 103552.
5. Wang G, Guo S, Han L, Cekderi AB, Song X, Zhao Z. Asymptomatic COVID-19 CT image denoising method based on wavelet transform combined with improved PSO[J]. Biomed Signal Process Control. 2022;76: 103707.
6. Sahba F, Venetsanopoulos A. A fuzzy approach for contrast enhancement of mammography breast images[M]. Adv. Comput. Biol. 2010.
7. Wu S, Yu S, Yang Y, Xie Y. Feature and contrast enhancement of mammographic image based on multiscale analysis and morphology[J]. Comput Math Methods Med. 2013;2013: 716948.
8. Malali HE, Assir A, Bhateja V, Mouhsen A, Harmouchi M. A contrast enhancement model for X-ray mammograms using modified local s-curve transformation based on multi-objective optimization[J]. IEEE Sens J. 2021;21(10):11543–54.
9. Wang Y, Jin Z, Wang Y. Research progress in fine structure enhancement methods of medical images[J]. J Biomed Eng. 2018;35(04):651–5 (in Chinese).
10. Liu L, Jia Z, Yang J, Kasabov N. A medical image enhancement method using adaptive thresholding in NSCT domain combined unsharp masking[J]. Int J Imaging Syst Technol. 2015;25(3):199–205.
11. Phophalia A, Mitra SK. Rough set based bilateral filter design for denoising brain MR images[J]. Appl Soft Comput. 2015;33:1–14.
12. Chaira T. An improved medical image enhancement scheme using type II fuzzy set[J]. Appl Soft Comput. 2014;25:293–308.
13. Bhardwaj A, Singh M. A novel approach of medical image enhancement based on Wavelet transform[J]. Comput. Sci. 2012.
14. Moreno R, Smedby Ö. Gradient-based enhancement of tubular structures in medical images[J]. Med Image Anal. 2015;26(1):19–29.
15. Mridha MF, Hamid MA, Monowar MM, Keya AJ, Ohi AQ, Islam MR, Kim JM. A comprehensive survey on deep-learning-based breast cancer diagnosis[J]. Cancers(Basel). 2021;13(23):6116.
16. Rouhi R, Jafari M, Kasaei S, Keshavarzian P. Benign and malignant breast tumors classification based on region growing and CNN segmentation[J]. Expert Syst Appl. 2015;42(3):990–1002.
17. Al-antari MA, Al-masni MA, Park SU, Park J, Metwally MK, Kadah YM, Han SM, Kim TS. An automatic computer-aided diagnosis system for breast cancer in digital mammograms via deep belief network[J]. J Med Biol Eng. 2018;38:443–56.
18. Ting FF, Tan YJ, Sim KS. Convolutional neural network improvement for breast cancer classification[J]. Expert Syst Appl. 2019;120:103–15.
19. Chougrad H, Zouaki H, Alheyane O. Deep convolutional neural networks for breast cancer screening[J]. Comput Methods Programs Biomed. 2018;157:19–30.
20. Li C, Xu J, Liu Q, Zhou Y, Mou L, Pu Z, Xia Y, Zheng H, Wang S. Multi-view mammographic density classification by dilated and attention-guided residual learning[J]. IEEE/ACM Trans Comput Biol Bioinf. 2021;18:1003–13.
21. Muduli D, Dash R, Majhi B. Automated breast cancer detection in digital mammograms: a moth flame optimization based ELM approach [J]. Biomed Signal Proc Control. 2020;59:101912.
22. Singh VK, Rashwan HA, Romani S, Akram F, Pandey N, Sarker MMK, Saleh A, Arenas M, Arquez M, Puig D, Torrents-Barrena J. Breast tumor segmentation and shape classification in mammograms using generative adversarial and convolutional neural network [J]. Expert Syst Appl. 2020;139:112855.

Chapter 4
Digital Twin Technology

4.1 Introduction

Current globalization trends demand complex and advanced information and communication technology systems. These demands have led to the advancement of digital infrastructure applied in research and production processes. The demands require new infrastructure such as networking of mobile devices, cloud infrastructure, data analytics algorithms and collective cloud services. This chapter explores the digital twin concept and how it is applied to healthcare.

Digital twin technology involves creating virtual simulation models of technical and physical assets that are maintained and changed by the information within a physical object (see Fig. 4.1). These models are quite dynamic and receive real-time readings of information from sensors of physical assets, sensors of control devices and the general environment. The models also take into consideration historical information obtained to adjust the parameters of the physical asset. These dynamic digital twin models enable the projection of technical objects into the digital platform. The systems update the measurements in real-time and are regularly updated on the new and old data using machine learning algorithms. The system's goal is to achieve the physical object's optimal operational capabilities through regular and dynamic updates. The digital twin system needs to continually learn and change its mode of operation based on inputs and updates by using methods such as artificial intelligence, machine learning, and neural networks. They can optimize operations of the physical assets through automatic monitoring of technical aspects, fault aspects, and prediction of the future status of operations.

The concept of the digital twin has been popularized by Grieves' conception of virtual and physical products. NASA has also brought about numerous digital twin technology contributions. The Air Force Research laboratory has also perfected the concepts through research and contributions. Siemens industries were the first industry player to apply digital twin technology in 2016. NASA defined the digital

S. Guo et al., *Advanced Technologies in Healthcare*,
https://doi.org/10.1007/978-981-99-9585-1_4

Fig. 4.1 Digital twin model

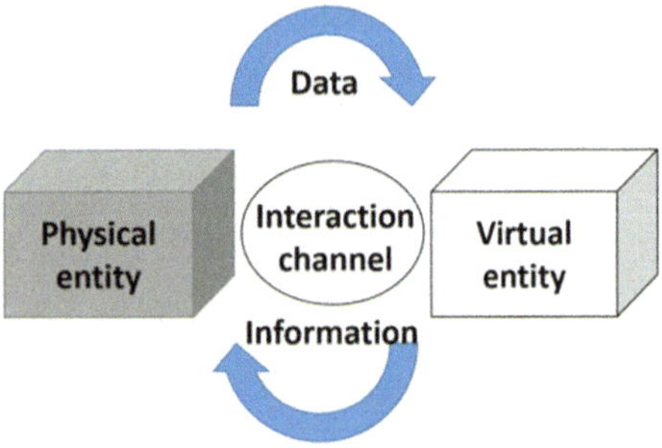

twin as an integration of multi-physics and probabilistic and multi-scale simulation of a vehicle or system that employed the most appropriate physical models, updated sensors, and fleeted history that mirror the operations of a corresponding twin. Grieves defined a digital twin as having three main operational parts: the physical asset in real space, the virtual products in virtual space and the connection of information that links the physical and virtual entities. It involved a virtual entity that mimicked the physical entity in the digital form to simulate the physical asset, which was a reflection of system performance, and could predict the future trends.

The technology links both the virtual and physical worlds, and the two models are becoming integrated, producing great effects and advantages. The digital twin technology has solved several information technology shortcomings and inadequacies, such as data acquisition, computer performance, algorithms and digital descriptions. The popularity of digital twin has witnessed its application in several fields with different users and different demands. The combination of digital twin and other technologies such as the Internet of Things has provided favorable cyber-physical interaction and data integration.

4.2 Components of Digital Twin Models

With three basic components of the real environment physical systems, the digital environment state and data linking these two states, digital twin is based on a five-dimensional model, which can be formulated as formula (4.1).

$$M_{\mathrm{DT}} = (\mathrm{PE}, \mathrm{VM}, \mathrm{Ss}, \mathrm{DD}, \mathrm{CN}), \tag{4.1}$$

where PE are physical entities, VM are virtual models, Ss are services, DD is digital twin data, and CN are connections. According to formula, the five-dimension digital twin model is shown in Fig. 4.2. As an enabling technology, digital twin is expected to become an integration of industry 4.0 for more widespread coverage, especially in healthcare to improve safety, cost saving and new products.

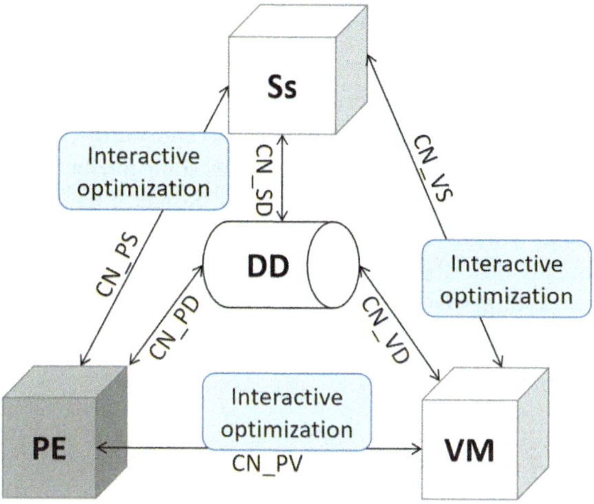

Fig. 4.2 Five-dimensional digital twin framework

4.2.1 Physical Entities in Digital Twin

Digital twin is to create the virtual models for physical entities in the digital way to simulate their behaviors. The physical entities are the foundation of digital twin technology. It can either be active processes, devices, products, physical systems or an organization. The digital twin models implement actions according to physical laws and deals in their environments. The physical entities can be divided into three levels: the unit level, the system level and the product level.

4.2.2 Virtual Models in Digital Twin

The three-dimensional geometric models that simulate the geometries, behaviors, dimensions, properties and rules of the corresponding physical entity are employed. Based on physical properties (e.g., speed, wear and force), physics model reflects the physical phenomena of the entities, such as the deformation, delamination, fracture and corrosion. Behavior model describes the behaviors (e.g., state transition, performance degradation and coordination) and responding mechanisms of the entities against changes in the external environment. The rule models equip digital twin with logical abilities such as reasoning, judgment, evaluation and autonomous decision-making, by following the rules extracted from historical data or come from domain experts.

4.2.3 Digital Twin Data

Digital twin data is a crucial driver of digital twin models. It engages a multi-temporal scale, heterogeneous, multi-source and multi-dimensional data. The data obtained from these physical entities, such as static attribute data or dynamic conditions, is key to running the digital twin models. Some of the user data is generated by the virtual twin, which reflects the results of the simulation. The data achieved from services mostly describes execution and invocation services. Another set of data is provided by domain experts from their pool of knowledge of the system, usually achieved by studying past or historical data.

4.2.4 Services in Digital Twin

Service is a key aspect of digital twins. Firstly, digital twin models give the users application services such as simulation, monitoring, verification, optimization and prognosis. Secondly, third-party services such as algorithm services, data services and knowledge services are fundamental in building functional digital twin models. Lastly, the operation of digital twin requires the continuous support of various platform services, which can accommodate customized software development, model building and service delivery.

4.2.5 Connections in Digital Twin

The virtual representatives are connected to their physical counterpart dynamically to facilitate advanced simulation, analysis and operations. There are connections among physical entities, virtual models, services and data to enable information to flow through the entire system and ensure ample collaboration among the four parts of the digital twin. There are six known connections in digital twin models: the connection between physical entities and virtual models (CN_PV), the connection between virtual models and services (CN_VS), the connection between virtual models and data (CN_VD), the connection between physical entities and data (CN_PD), the connection between physical entities and services (CN_PS) and the connection between services and data (CN_SD).

4.3 Conceptual Modeling of Digital Twin [1]

A digital twin is the systematic expression of the components, behaviors, and rules of a physical entity. Hence, this section presents an approach to the construction of a digital twin conceptual model that incorporates the improved TRIZ function modeling method guided by the five-dimensional framework. Starting with the functions of the modules, this section gradually decomposes functions, defines the executive components of each function and illustrates the physical entity modules. Concurrently, based on the conceptual model of the physical entity, a conceptual model of each module is constructed via its function and an analysis thereof. From the interactions between modules, the initial conceptual structure can be gradually improved to create an accurate conceptual digital twin model. The specific construction process is shown in Fig. 4.3. Detailed steps are as follows:

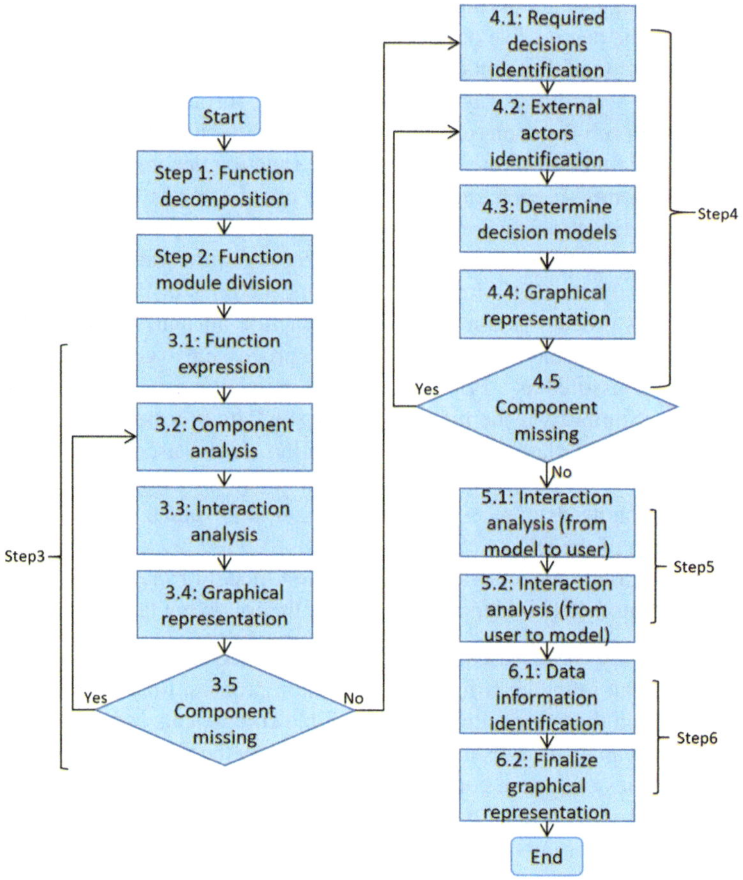

Fig. 4.3 Proposed conceptual modeling of digital twin

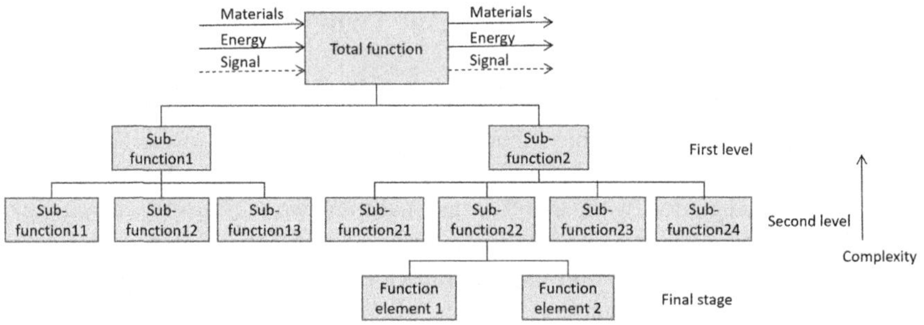

Fig. 4.4 Function analysis process

Step 1: Perform a function analysis to identify and decompose the digital twin's functions. First, designers are to identify the initial input and final output of the model according to energy, materials and signals. The input and output of the model can be analyzed from the perspective of the user's need or expectation. Based on the input and output of the model, its total function can be determined. The model can then be decomposed according to its realization process, through which designers can determine which sub-functions are required to realize the total function. This is then used as the total function of the second level of function decomposition. Designers continue to decompose each sub-function and use the forms of sub-functions to represent them. This process of analysis ends when the total function is decomposed into function elements. The function analysis process is illustrated in Fig. 4.4.

Step 2: Classify functions into corresponding modules of the five-dimensional framework. This process is completed using function attributes. If a function acts directly on the external environment without data processing to generate instructions, the function is classified as a PE function. Data collection can also be classified as a PE function. Similarly, if the function focuses on data processing and instruction generation, it can be classified as a VM function. If the user is involved in the realization process of the function, the function should be classified as part of the Ss. If the function needs to receive relevant data or store data temporarily, it can be classified as part of the DD.

Step 3: Construct the expanded TRIZ function model of the PE as the basis for the conceptual model. This step is composed of the following tasks:

(1) Function expression. Based on the results of the decomposition of the function, designers can refine each function realization process. Function actuators can be found and the composition of the tangible components can be determined.
(2) Component analysis. This is carried out to classify the tangible components into the categories of system components, super-system components or product. If the component is a fixed part of the system, it is a system component. If the component exists outside the system but interacts with it, it is a super-system component. The system's target object is the product.
(3) Interaction analysis. Based on results of the function analysis, designers can analyze a given component's role in the model's operation process, clarifying

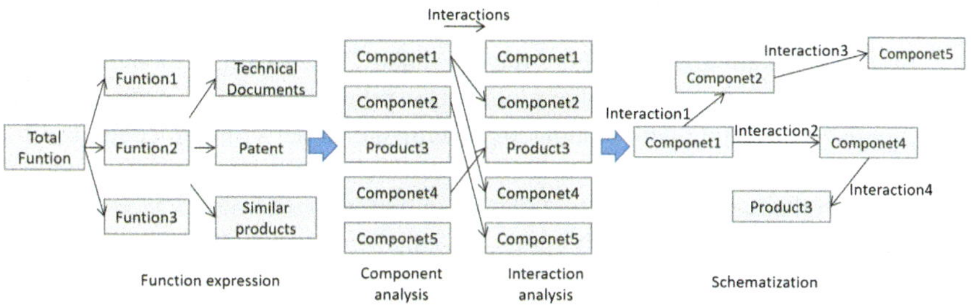

Fig. 4.5 Modeling process for the physical entity (PE)

the interactions between different components. Designers can define the type of a specific interaction between two components via their outputs. The concrete form of the outputs, such as energy and signal, represents the interaction between them. If the interaction contributes to the model's operation, it is a standard effect. If it is not conducive to the model's operation, it is a harmful effect. If it has a certain deviation from the standard effect, without affecting system operation, it is an insufficient or excessive effect.

(4) Schematizing components and their interactions. Components are expressed using schemata of the system components, super-system components and product. The interactions of different components are expressed using various types of arrows. Their interactions are also briefly described. An initial conceptual digital twin model is thusly established.

(5) Checking the PE model. According to the results of the component analysis, the conceptual PE model is checked to ensure that it includes all of the necessary components. This construction process is shown in Fig. 4.5.

Step 4: The VM completes the data analysis to generate corresponding instructions and optimize the PE's operation. The initial conceptual model needs to be subsequently improved according to the VM's informational characteristics. The specific process is as follows:

(1) Identifying the decision model. The VM analyzes data from either the environment or other digital twins to optimize the model's operation. The decision model is needed during this process in order to conduct the analysis. The type of the decision model and other relevant information can be determined using the required control instructions.

(2) Identifying the components that interact with the model. Via the decision model, the VM analyzes real-time data and generates corresponding instructions. When designers modify the initial conceptual model based on the VM, the interactions between the model and other objects in the environment should be considered. Designers can analyze the data collected by the PE and the usage scenarios to determine possibly influential objects in the environment. In addition, to form a digital twin system, or ensure its optimal function output, different models may interact with each other. Therefore, designers need to consider whether such

corresponding interactions exist. Other digital twin models can be represented by super-system components of the expanded TRIZ function model to further modify the existing conceptual model during the schematizing process.

(3) Identifying the judgment module. In general, the model's function outputs differ depending on its usage scenario. The specific conditions may occur under a function that can then be refined based on the influence of the given scenario. According to the trigger conditions, designers can extract behavior rules, with each rule corresponding to a specific function. These rules are then used to evaluate the modules to improve the initial conceptual digital twin model. After defining a specific form of module evaluation, designers can use the interaction form of the TRIZ function model to express the outputs according to different rules.

(4) Verifying the model with all interactive objects.

Step 5: The Ss can provide some guidance for interactions between users and the digital twin model. In order to ensure the accuracy of the modeling process, the conceptual model must be improved based on the Ss with respect to the following two aspects.

(1) The interaction between the model and the user (from model to user), including interaction analysis to identify the type of service fed back by the digital twin model to improve the super-system module of the initial conceptual model, clarifying personalized service and identifying the interaction mode in which the model feeds information back to users.

(2) The interaction between the user and the model (from user to model), including interaction analysis to determine the feedback between users and Ss, presenting the way to feed user-relevant information back to the model if the corresponding information feedback exists, and clarifying behavioral feedback. This construction process is shown in Fig. 4.6.

Step 6: Identify data-related information. Despite being required to store the model's original data, the DD also needs to store derived data related to function execution during the product's life cycle to ensure real-time prediction and optimization. The component included by the PE is the data collection port. If the need for data transmission exists, it is necessary to define the decision model with support from data and to determine the type of this data via the components' characteristics. The VM mainly conducts data analyses and generates relevant instructions. Therefore, based on the types and principles of the decision model, the data input and corresponding output (data/instructions) can be analyzed to determine the data-related information. For the Ss, designers analyze users to establish information that may contribute to the modified design of the digital twin. After the data-related information of each module is defined, the content can be supplemented in the schemata of each component to ensure the existing conceptual model's accuracy.

By following the above steps, the conceptual digital twin model comprises a comprehensive embodiment of components, behaviors and rules, all of which are fully represented by the components and the interactions among them. The proposed

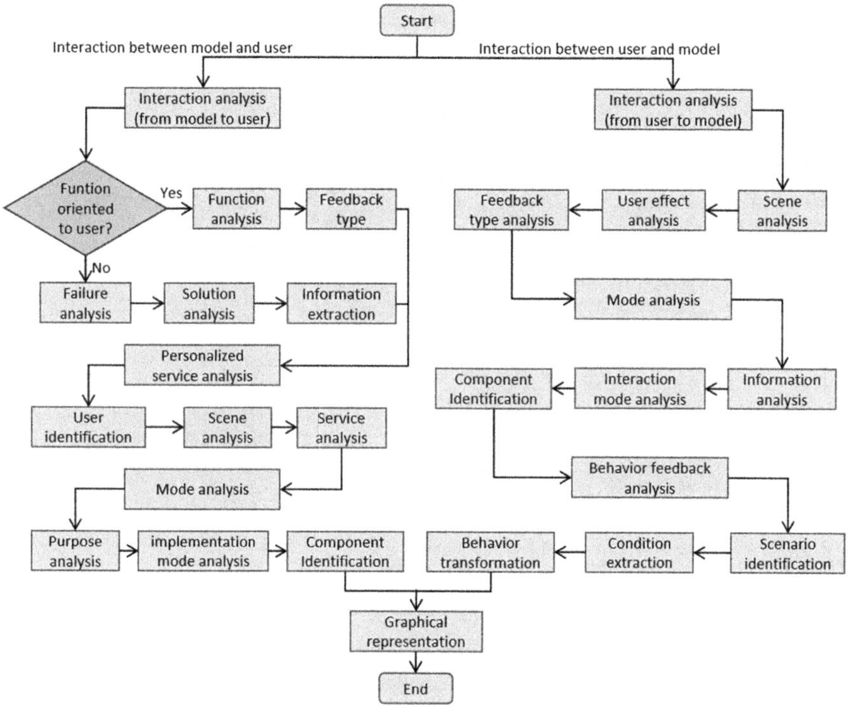

Fig. 4.6 Modeling process for the services module (Ss)

method thus provides guidance for the construction of a digital twin model that considers various factors in the process of constructing a conceptual digital twin model.

4.4 Technologies Employed in Digital Twin Models [2]

According to the five-dimensional model, as shown in Fig. 4.7, a variety of enabling technologies are required to support different modules of digital twin. For the physical entity, the full understanding for the physical world is a prerequisite for digital twin, including dynamics, structural mechanics, electromagnetism, materials science, control theory and more. Combined with the sensing and measurement technologies, the physical entities and processes are mapped to the virtual space to make the models more accurate and closer to the reality. For the virtual model, various modeling technologies are essential, including visualization technologies for real-time monitoring, verification, validation and accreditation (VV&A) technologies, optimization algorithms, simulation and retrospective technologies for rapid diagnosis and model evolution technologies for driving the model update. During the

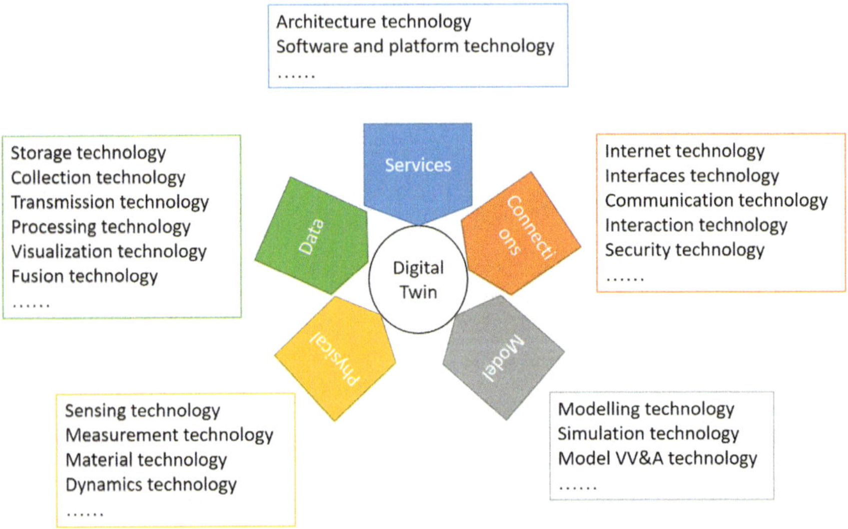

Fig. 4.7 Framework of enabling technologies for digital twin

operation of digital twin, a huge volume of data is generated, which involves data collection, transmission, storage, processing, fusion and visualization. To deliver digital twin-related services, it requires application software, platform architecture technology, service oriented architecture (SoA) technologies and knowledge technologies. Finally, the connection involves Internet technologies, interaction technologies, cyber-security technologies, interface technologies, communication protocols, etc.

4.4.1 Enabling Technologies for Cognizing and Controlling Physical World

The creation of virtual models is based on the entities in the physical world, as well as their key internal interaction logic and external relationships. To create high-fidelity models, it is imperative to cognize the physical world and perceive data. As shown in Fig. 4.8, the first step to reflect the physical world is to measure the parameters. The existing measurement technologies include laser measurement, image recognition measurement, conversion measurement and micro/nano-level precision measurement. In addition, sophisticated digital twins continuously pull real-time sensor and system data to represent a near real-time as-is state of physical entities. Furthermore, digital twin serves to improve the performance of physical entities in the physical world. When the entities in physical world carry out the intended

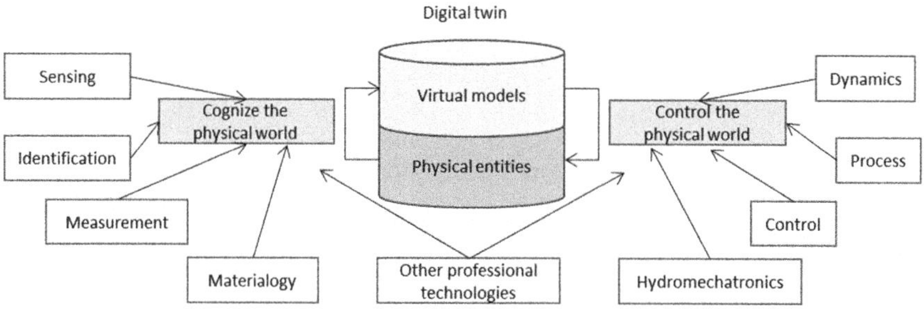

Fig. 4.8 Enabling technologies for cognizing and controlling physical world

functions, the energy is controlled by control system to drive their actuators to accurately complete the specified actions. This process involves power technologies, drive systems, process technologies and control technologies.

Digital twin applications call for new technologies (such as big data analytics and machine vision) to better perceive the physical world. For now, it is recommended to use image recognition and laser measurement technologies to measure the parameters of the physical world, and use electrical control, programmable control, embedded control and network control technologies to control the physical world, as well as use big data analysis technologies to mine the implicit laws and knowledge.

4.4.2 Enabling Technologies for Digital Twin Modeling

Modeling refers to the process of representing a physical entity in digital forms that can be processed, analyzed and managed by computers. Modeling is arguably the cornerstone of digital twin, as shown in Fig. 4.9, digital twin-related modeling involves geometric modeling, physical modeling, behavioral modeling and rule modeling.

Geometric modeling describes a physical entity in terms of its geometric shape, topological information, embodiment and appearance with appropriate data structures, which are suitable for computer information conversion and processing. Geometric modeling includes wireframe modeling, surface modeling and solid modeling. Besides, to increase the sense of reality, developers create appearance texture effects with bitmaps that represent the surface details of the entity. Physical modeling adds information such as accuracy information, material information and assembly information. Feature modeling includes interactive feature definition, automatic feature recognition and feature-based design. Behavioral modeling describes various behaviors of a physical entity to fulfill functions, respond to changes, interact with others, adjust internal operations, maintain health, etc. The simulation of physical behaviors is a complex process that involves multiple models, such as problem modeling, state modeling, dynamics modeling, evaluation modeling. These models

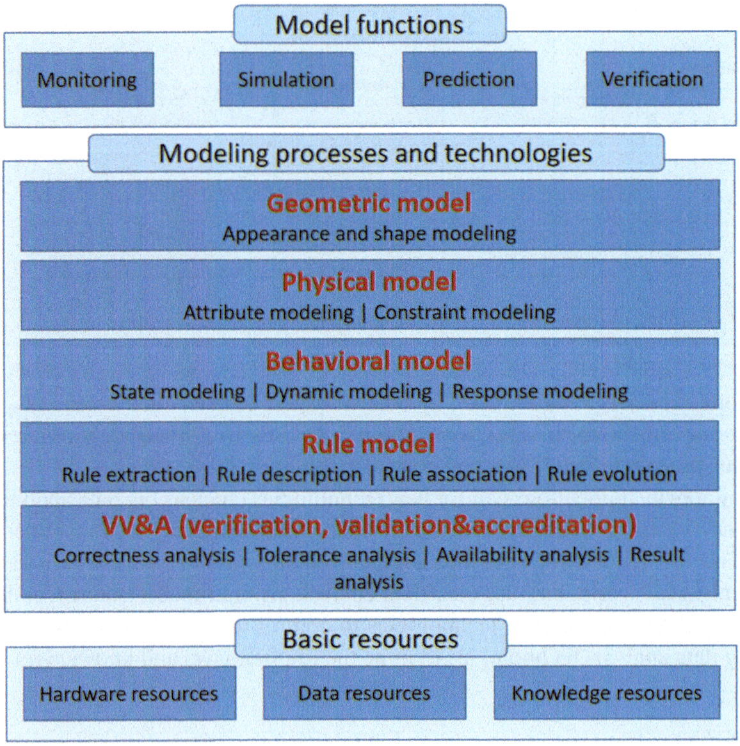

Fig. 4.9 Enabling technologies for modeling

can be developed based on finite state machines, Markov chains, ontology-based modeling methods, etc.

Rule modeling describes the rules extracted from historical data, expert knowledge and predefined logic. The rules equip the virtual model with an ability to reason, judge, evaluate, optimize and predict. Rule modeling involves rule extraction, rule description, rule association and rule evolution. Rule extraction involves both symbolic methods (e.g., decision tree and rough set theory) and connectionist methods (e.g., neural network). Rule description involves methods such as logical notation, production representation, frame representation, object-oriented representation, semantic web notation, XML-based representation, ontology representation, etc. Rule association involves methods such as category association, diagnostic/inferential association, cluster association, behavior association and attribute association. Rule evolution includes application evolution and periodic evolution. Application evolution means the process of adjusting and updating the rules based on feedback obtained from the application process, and periodic evolution means the process of regularly evaluating the effectiveness of current rules over a certain period of time (the time varies depending on the application).

Model VV&A can improve model accuracy and simulation confidence. Model VV&A involves both static methods and dynamic methods. Static methods are used to evaluate the static aspect of modeling and simulation, including grammatical analysis, semantic analysis, structural analysis, causal maps, control analysis, etc. Dynamic methods are used to validate the dynamic aspects of modeling and simulation, including black box test, white box test, execution tracking, regression testing, statistical technique and graphical comparison.

The current modeling technologies focus on the construction of geometric and physical models. It remains a challenge to integrate various models with different dimensions, different spatial scales and different time scales. Modeling should be optimized for multi-objective and full-performance, to reach high accuracy, reliability and reproduce both dynamic and static characteristics. Moreover, combined with the historical usage, maintenance and upgrade data, various digital twin models can be progressively optimized through Bayesian, machine learning, as well as other data mining methods and optimization algorithms.

4.4.3 Enabling Technologies for Digital Twin Data Management

As illustrated in Fig. 4.10, the whole data lifecycle includes data collection, transmission, storage, processing, fusion and visualization. Barcodes, QR codes, radio frequency identification devices (RFID), cameras, sensor and other IoT technologies are widely used for hardware data collection. Software data can be collected through software application programming interfaces (APIs), and open database interfaces. Network data can be collected from the Internet through web crawlers, search engine and public APIs. Data transmission technologies include wire and wireless transmissions. Wire transmission technologies include twisted-pair cable transmission, symmetric cable transmission, coaxial cable transmission, fiber optic transmission, etc. Wireless transmission includes short-range and long-distance technologies. The widely used short-range wireless technologies include Zig-Bee, Bluetooth, Wi-Fi, Ultra-Wideband (UWB) and Near Field Communication (NFC). Long-distance wireless technologies include GPRS/CDMA, digital radio, spread spectrum microwave, wireless bridge, satellite communication, etc.

Data storage is to store the collected data for further processing, analysis and management. Due to the increasing volume and heterogeneity of multi-source digital twin data, big data storage technologies, such as distributed file storage (DFS), NoSQL database, NewSQL database and cloud storage, are drawing growing attention. DFS enables many hosts to access shared files and directories simultaneously over the network. NoSQL is characterized by the ability to scale horizontally to cope with massive data. NewSQL denotes new scalable and high-performance databases, which not only has storage and management capability for massive data, but also implements replication and failback by using redundant machines. Data processing

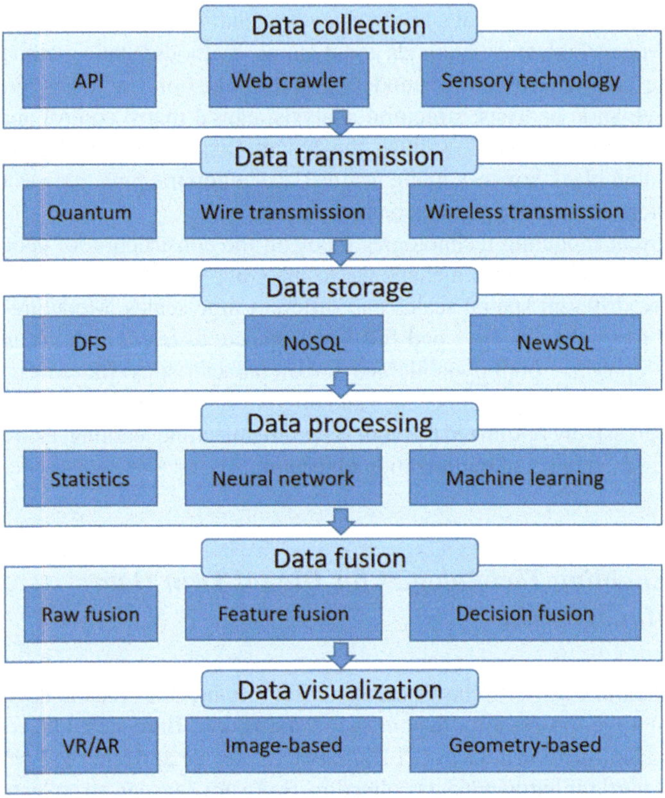

Fig. 4.10 Enabling technologies for digital twin data management

means extracting useful information from a large volume of incomplete, unstructured, noisy, fuzzy and random raw data. Firstly, data is carefully preprocessed to remove redundant, irrelevant, misleading, duplicate and inconsistent data. The relevant technologies include data cleaning, data compression, data smoothing, data reduction, data transformation, etc. Next, the pre-processed data is analyzed through statistical methods, neural network methods, etc. Relevant statistical methods and neural network methods are shown in Fig. 4.11.

Data fusion copes with multi-source data through synthesis, filtering, correlation and integration. Data fusion includes raw-data-level fusion, feature-level fusion and decision-level fusion. Data fusion methods include random methods and artificial intelligence. Random methods (e.g., classical reasoning, weighted average method, Kalman filtering, Bayesian estimation and Dempster-Shafer evidence reasoning) are applicable for all three levels of data fusion. Artificial intelligence methods (e.g., fuzzy set theory, rough set theory, neural network, wavelet theory and support vector machine) are applicable for the feature-level and decision-level data fusions. Data visualization serves to present data analysis results in a straightforward, intuitive and

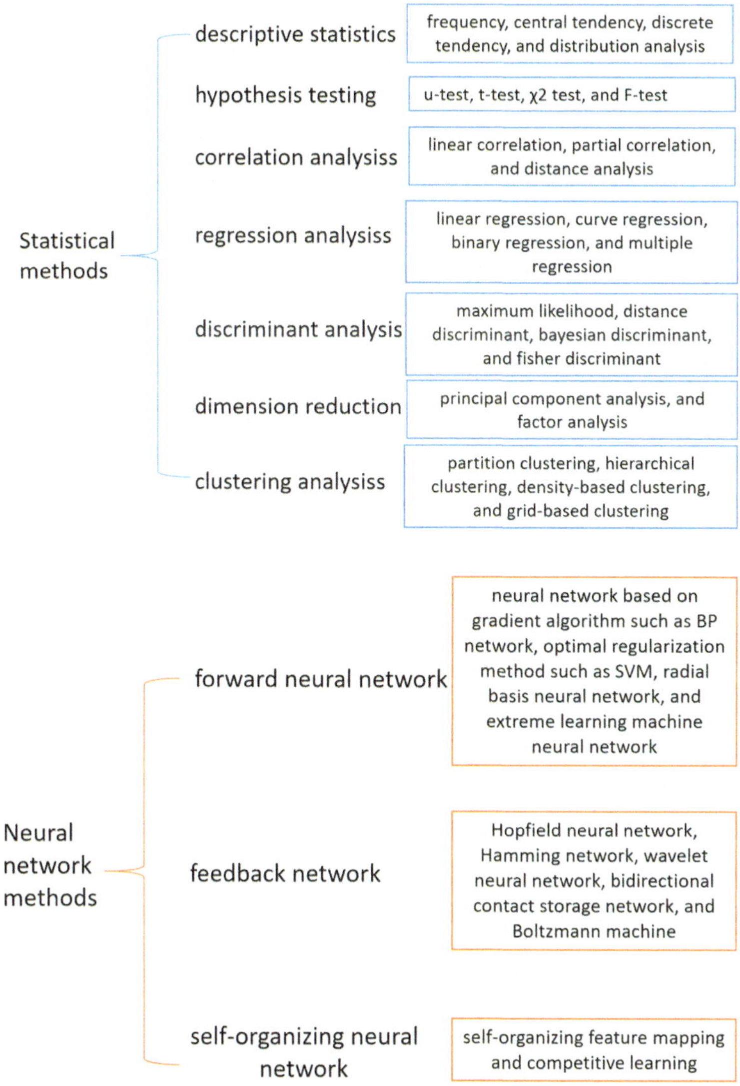

Fig. 4.11 Relevant statistical and neural network methods

interactive manner. According to the principle of its visualization, these methods can be divided into geometry-based technologies, pixel-oriented technologies, icon-based technologies, layer-based technologies, image-based technologies, etc.

As the volume of data continues to increase, the existing data technologies are bound to advance. Now, the recommendation of key technologies for data lifecycle management includes sensors and other IoT technologies for data collection, 5G or even 6G technology for data transmission, NewSQL technology for data storage, edge-cloud architecture computing technology for data processing and artificial intelligence technology for data fusion.

4.4.4 Enabling Technologies for Digital Twin Services

As shown in Fig. 4.12, digital twin integrates multiple disciplines to achieve advanced monitoring, simulation, diagnosis and prognosis. Monitoring requires computer graphics, image processing, 3D rendering, graphics engine, virtual-reality synchronization technologies, etc. Simulation involves structural simulation, mechanics (e.g., fluid dynamics, solid mechanics, thermodynamics and kinematics) simulation, electronic circuit simulation, control simulation, process simulation, virtual test simulation, etc. Diagnosis and prognosis are based on data analysis, which involves statistical theory, machine learning, neural network, fuzzy theory, fault tree, etc.

Some hardware and software resources and even knowledge can be encapsulated into services. The lifecycle of resource services can be divided into three stages: service generation, service management and on-demand use of services. Service generation technologies include resource perception and assessing, resource virtualization, resource encapsulation technologies, etc. Service management technologies include service searching, matching, collaboration, comprehensive utility evaluation, quality of service (QoS), scheduling, fault tolerance technologies, etc. On-demand use technologies consisted of transaction and business management technologies, etc. Knowledge services involve the process of knowledge capture, storage, sharing, reuse, etc. Common technologies for knowledge capturing include association rule mining, statistical methods, artificial neural network, decision tree, rough set method, case-based reasoning method, etc. Knowledge storage, sharing and reuse are implemented in the form of services.

Resource and knowledge services, application services can be managed through the industrial IoT platform. The platform provides some supporting functions such as service publishing, querying, searching, smart matching and recommendation, online communication, online contracting, service evaluation, etc. Platform-related technologies include platform architecture, organization mode, operation and maintenance management, security technologies, etc.

4.4.5 Enabling Technologies for Connections in Digital Twin

In the connections in digital twin, the communication interfaces and protocol technologies, human–computer interaction technologies, as well as security technologies should be pay more attention.

As shown in Fig. 4.13, based on the real-time data exchange through CN_PV, not only the running state of the physical entities is reflected dynamically in the virtual world, but also the analysis results of the virtual models are sent back to

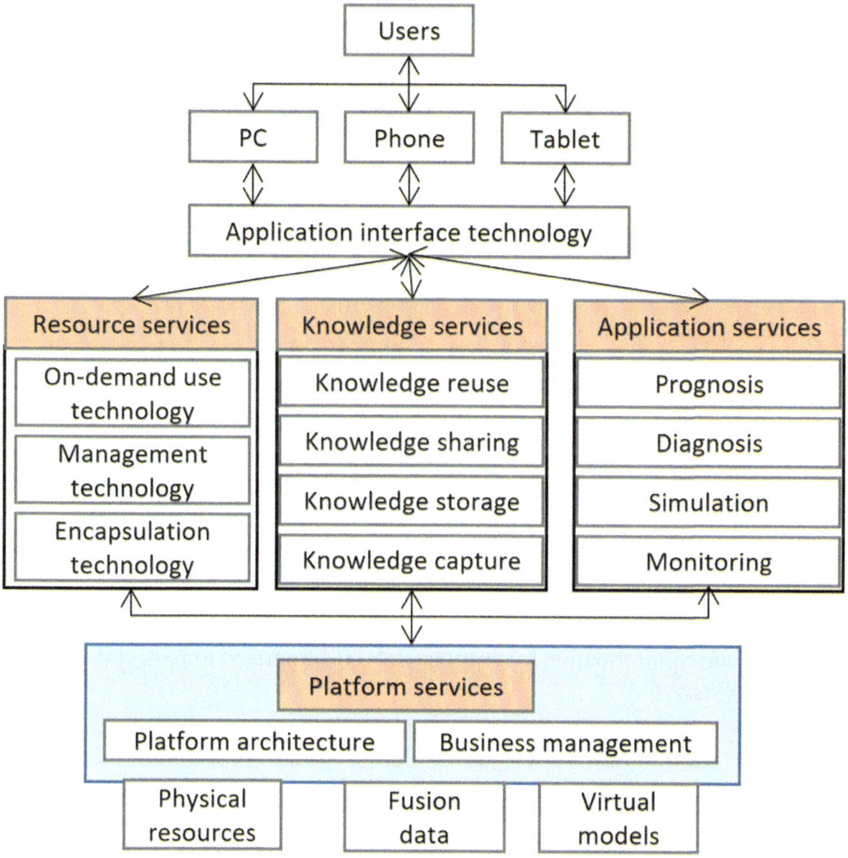

Fig. 4.12 Enabling technologies for digital twin services

control the physical entities. Through CN_PD, digital twin is used to manage the entire product lifecycle, which laid data foundation for analysis, prediction, quality tracing and product planning. Through CN_PS, services (e.g., monitoring, diagnostics and prognosis) are linked to physical entities to receive data and feed the service outcome back. Therefore, RFID, sensor, wireless sensor network and other IoT technologies are necessary. Data exchange requires communication technology, unified communication interfaces and protocol technologies, including protocol parsing and conversion, interface compatibility, common gateway interface, etc. Given many different models, CN_VD needs communication, interfaces, protocols and standard technologies to ensure smooth data interaction between virtual models and data. Similarly, the connections between services and virtual models (CN_VS) as well as data (CN_SD) also require communication interface, protocol, standard technologies and collaboration technologies. Finally, security technologies (e.g., device security,

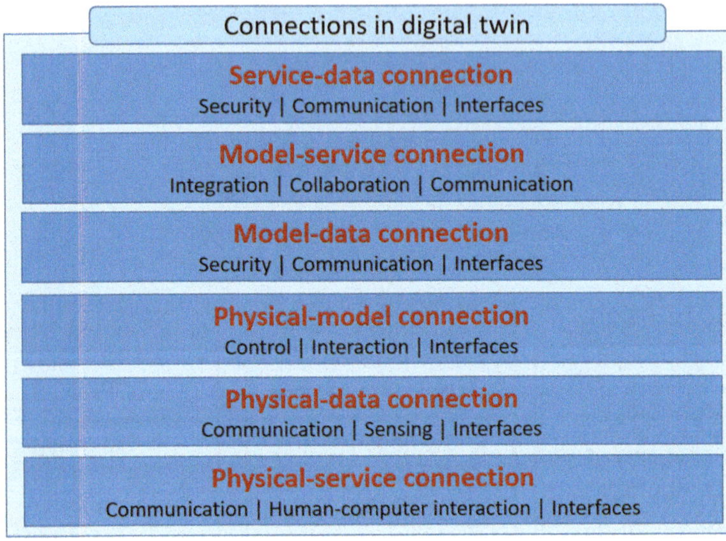

Fig. 4.13 Enabling technologies for connections

network security, information security) must be incorporated to protect the security of digital twins.

4.5 Digital Twin Technology in Healthcare

Over the years, the digital twin application is key to the growth of high-tech healthcare systems. Impossible procedures are slowly becoming possible with AI and IoT in diagnosis, prognosis and treatment. The application could include the following aspects:

- Digital twin systems are currently used to undertake novel drug trials for side effects, efficacy, safety and dosage. This simulation will eliminate the need to use human beings and animals as experimental subjects.
- Digital twin is employed to plan and execute complex surgical procedures. Digital twin technology has improved this through real-time simulations that project the specific patient situation.
- In the coming years, patient's body will be fitted with a digital twin system that gives a real-time analysis of its vitals to physicians.
- In combination with AI, digital twin can predict malaise and disease based on information that is relayed in real-time or from the patient's historical data.
- Digital twin ensures safety by virtualizing a hospital system to assess the safety of tests and environments.

- Digital twin is applied in the predictive maintenance and repair of hospital equipment by lowering their stalling due to abrupt breakdowns.

Healthcare is very dependent on research. Biomedical scientists have employed digital twin technology to identify gaps that require research. These insights empower medical scientists to have a wide horizon of thought in helping to achieve medical solutions through predictive maintenance of research, aspects to analyze results and a discovery. In this section, the digital twin in orthopedics, cardiovascular disease, chronic disease, pharmacy and others are discussed.

4.5.1 Orthopedics

In order to make up for the shortcomings of traditional biomechanical analysis methods in dynamic observation, He et al. [3] carried out the first attempt of the digital twin in orthopedics (Fig. 4.14). They built a shape-performance integrated digital twin body to predict the biomechanical properties of the real lumbar spine under different human postures with the help of customized information collection of the lumbar spine bones of a specific experimenter. Based on human motion capture technology, the real-time motion posture and spatial position of the human body were obtained. The lumbar posture of the corresponding human body was calculated according to the wearable virtue reality device and a small amount of sensor data. Using the information of the inverse kinematics system and combined with the finite element method, the digital twin body of the lumbar spine was established, so as to realize various motion postures of the human body. The AI model performed real-time calculations based on the obtained posture information and the results were fused with the virtual lumbar spine by visualization. In addition, the biomechanical properties of the lumbar spine were evaluated and predicted in real-time and achieved the purpose of real-time monitoring and prediction. Finally, a three-dimensional (3D) virtual-reality system was developed with the help of Unity3D software to record the real-time biomechanical performance of the lumbar spine, which could provide a new and effective method of real-time planning in the field of spine treatments. Based on the method for constructing the digital twin, they have realized the real-time prediction of the intradiskal pressure and the facet contact force, as well as dynamic interaction and connection between physical space and digital space.

To optimize surgical trauma procedures and improve decision-making in post-operative management, Aubert et al. [4] created the digital twin of a patient's fracture and modeled four stabilization methods. Repeated fracture risks were evaluated regarding the volume of bone with stress above the local yield strength and regarding the interfragmentary strains.

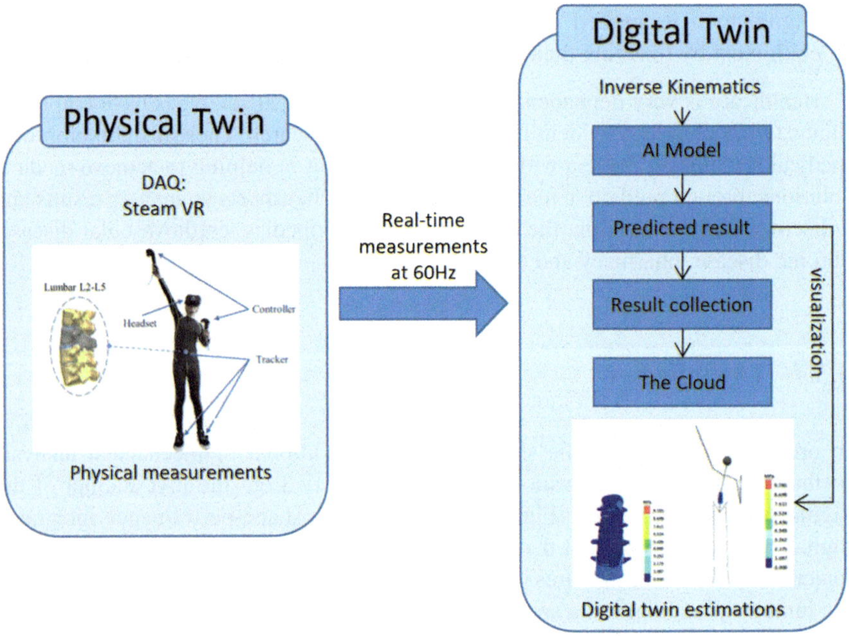

Fig. 4.14 Toward a shape-performance integrated digital twin for lumbar spine analysis

4.5.2 Cardiovascular Disease

The application of the digital twin in the cardiovascular system includes the establishment of digital heart models and precise treatment of cardiovascular diseases. Philips [5] developed the personalized digital twin model based on the unique CT images of the heart, which were obtained before the surgical procedure. The tool can provide real-time 3D positioning services to help surgeons locate and select equipment during surgery. Chakshu et al. [6] used a recurrent neural network and proposed a methodology for inverse analysis to enable the cardiovascular digital twin, which can perform inverse analysis with high accuracy. The easy-accessible arteries blood pressure waveforms such as radial or carotid arteries were used as input to calculate aortic blood pressure waveforms inversely with the help of deep learning methods and long short-term memory (LSTM) cells. The inverse analysis method made it possible to develop an active digital twin that can continuously monitor and prevent the development or further deterioration of medical conditions. The inverse analysis system built by this way was applied to the detection of abdominal aortic aneurysm (AAA) and its severity using neural networks (see Fig. 4.15). In summary, a deep neural network was first used to determine waveforms at various locations of a blood flow network and then an addition neural network of a different configuration was employed to analyze AAA diameter.

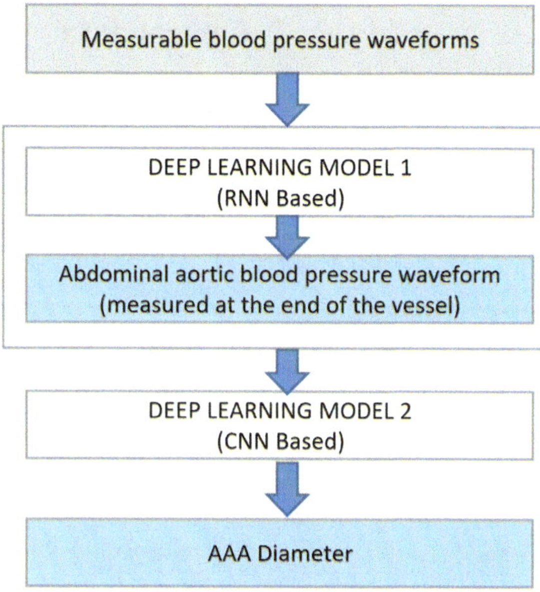

Fig. 4.15 LSTM-based inverse analysis and AAA classification

Personalized computer models of cardiac function, referred to as cardiac digital twins, are envisioned to play an important role in clinical precision therapies of cardiovascular diseases. A major obstacle hampering clinical translation involves the significant computational costs involved in the personalization of biophysically detailed mechanistic models that requires the identification of high-dimensional parameter vectors. Jung et al. [7] established a personalized 3D electromechanics (EM) model by calibration to clinical cavity pressure data from patients treated for aortic coarctation, and generated a high-fidelity model at the cellular scale. Figure 4.16 shows the integrated workflow for building digital twins of cardiac electromechanics. In the first step, active mechanical behavior in a given 3D EM model was represented by a purely phenomenological, low-fidelity model, which was personalized at the organ scale by calibration to clinical cavity pressure data. Then, in the second step, median traces of nodal cellular active stress, intracellular calcium concentration, and fiber stretch were generated and utilized to personalize the desired high-fidelity model at the cellular scale using a 0D model of cardiac EM.

4.5.3 Chronic Disease

The application of the digital twin in healthcare is mainly focused on chronic disease management. For example, in neurocritical care (NCC), current digital technologies focus on interpreting electroencephalogram (EEG), monitoring intracranial pressure, and simulating prognosis. It can interpret EEG by helping annotation tracking,

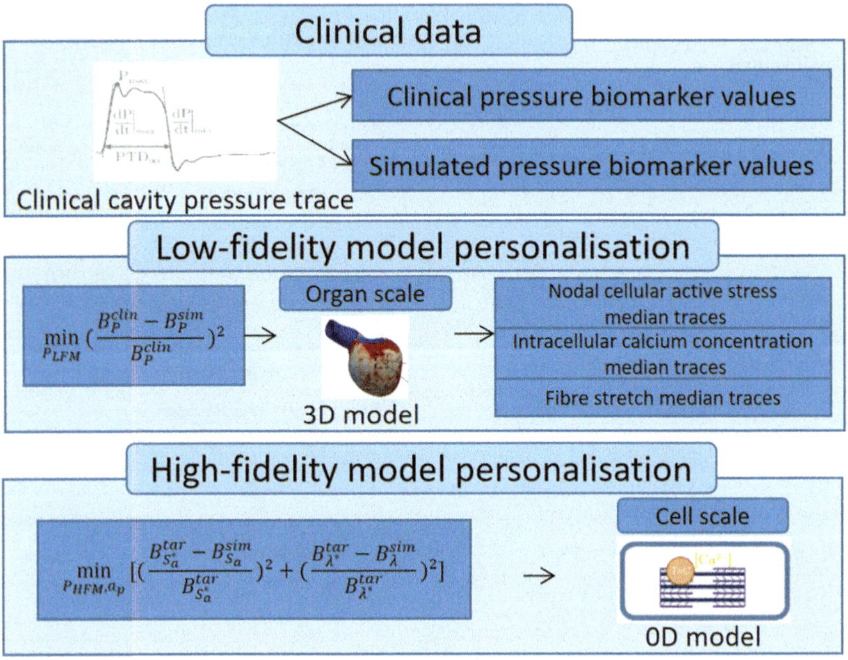

Fig. 4.16 Conceptual illustration of the two-step multi-fidelity approach for personalizing biophysically detailed active mechanics models

detecting seizures, and identifying brain activation in unresponsive patients [8]. Illustrations of how digital twin models could be conceptually built for application in NCC are shown in Fig. 4.17. In applying this model to a patient with ischemic stroke, for example, factors such as blood pressure, glucose levels, securing an airway, and giving anticoagulation, thrombolytics or opiate medication are all actionable factors that can be input into the AI model. These actions will affect certain semi-actionable factors and the overarching concept in the digital twin AI model such as hemorrhage, edema, aspiration, and, ultimately, ischemic stroke, all connected by Bayesian networks. With this digital twin of the patient, trainees will be able to test different interventions and get real-time feedback on the effects of their intervention without ever having to worry about potential harm to the actual patient.

In an artificial pancreas model for patients with type 1 diabetes, mathematical models of human glucose metabolism and data algorithms that simulate insulin delivery are customized into the patient-specific digital twin model, which can continuously calculate insulin requirements and regulate blood insulin concentrations [9]. Li et al. presented a scalable framework for modeling and prioritizing upstream regulators (URs) for biomarker- and drug discovery among dynamic changes in the digital twins for seasonal allergic rhinitis (SAR) [10]. They started with SAR as a disease model, by analyzing of in vitro allergen-stimulated peripheral blood mononuclear

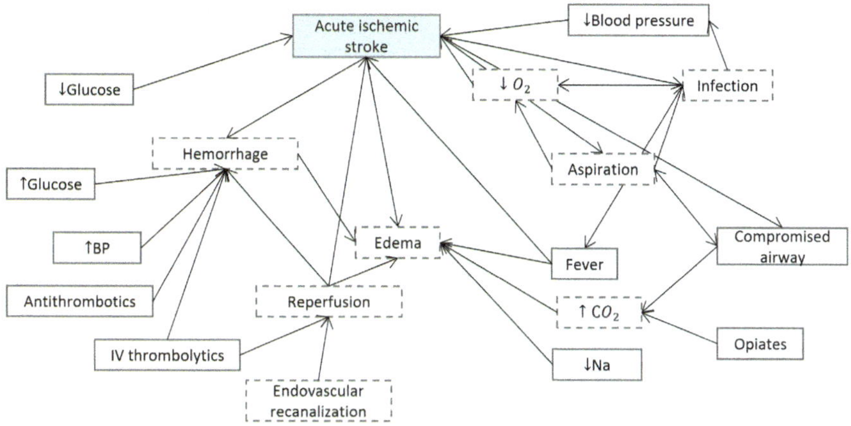

Fig. 4.17 A directed acyclic graph for stroke patients that link concepts through Bayesian networks built from an underlying understanding of disease processes (Blue boxes represent concepts, black solid lines represent actionable factors, dashed black lines represent semi-actionable factors, arrows represent Bayesian connections between different variables)

cells (PBMC) from SAR patients. Time-series single-cell RNA-sequencing (scRNA-seq) data of these cells were used to construct multi-cellular network models (MNMs) at each time point of molecular interactions between cell types. They hypothesized that predicted molecular interactions between cell types in the MNMs could be traced to find an UR gene, at an early time point. They performed bioinformatic and functional studies of the MNMs to develop a scalable framework to prioritize UR genes (Fig. 4.18).

4.5.4 *Pharmacy*

Dassault Systèmes and the US Food and Drug Administration signed off in 2014 for a project named the SIMULIA Living Heart, which was the first study to look at the organ–drug interactions digitally [11]. This was a digital twin model simulating human hearts and has been validated by researchers or educators in the medical field. Here they presented a proof-of concept simulator for a four-chamber human heart model created from computed topography and magnetic resonance images. With this technology, doctors and pharmaceutical engineers could see the complex structure or the mobility of heart tissue, which would lead to personalized treatment in the future such as stenosis, regurgitation or prolapse of the aortic, pulmonary, tricuspid or mitral valve.

Takeda Pharmaceuticals has switched to the digital twin technology in production to deliver transformative therapies globally. By creating the digital twin models, it can shorten pharmaceutical processes and make realistic input–output predictions for

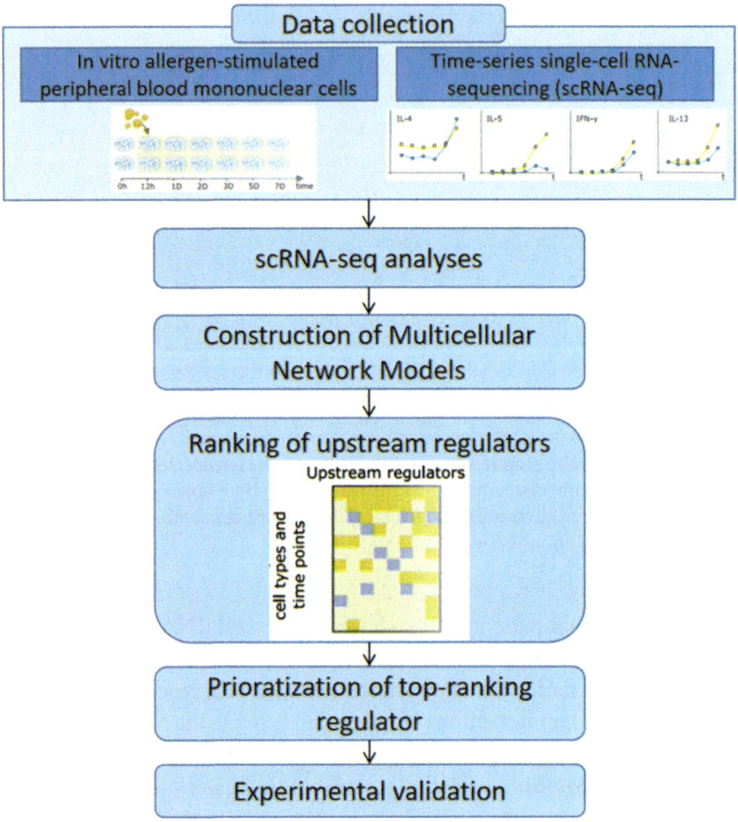

Fig. 4.18 A scalable framework for inferring UR genes on dynamic cellulome- and genome-wide scales

biochemical reactions. Atos and Siemens worked with the pharmaceutical industry to improve the manufacturing process through the physical digital twin models, which were created to overcome the difficulties in efficiency and production. It was currently tested to be successful and was supported by the IoT, AI and many other advanced technologies [9].

4.5.5 Others

Liu et al. [12] proposed a new concept of digital twin healthcare (DTH) in 2019, which was acted as a novel medical simulation method to provide robust, precise and effective medical services using technology combined with multi-disciplinary, multi-physics and multi-scale models. They proposed an effective, highly confidential and query-like healthcare monitoring plan based on the digital twin platform.

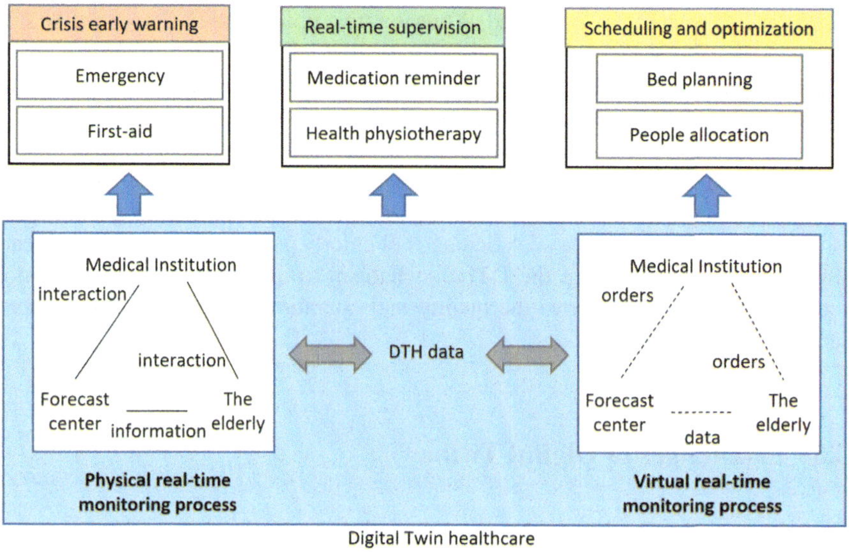

Fig. 4.19 Scenario of CloudDTH applications

The system consisted of three parts: physical object, virtual object and healthcare data. Each patient was connected to the digital twin, which could monitor his status and provide strong support in cloud healthcare services for the elderly. As shown in Fig. 4.19, in this application scenario, the cloud health system based on digital twin healthcare (CloudDTH) included external factors, elderly patients, healthcare institutions, corresponding mirror virtual model and DTH data. Below, the specific services of crisis early warning, real-time supervision and resources scheduling are discussed.

First, as a crisis early warning service, external environmental factors such as the temperature change, road surface status and wind speed; healthcare records data; and physical sensor data of elderly patients will be transferred to the virtual supervision process module. With the help of modeling methods based on the CloudDTH simulation service, a DTH simulation scenario will be constructed. After that, fast simulation can be done according to a virtual model, and the simulation results will be sent to the healthcare institution, elderly patients and their caregivers. Furthermore, dangerous events such as falling can be predicted through iteration of the virtual DTH model using machine learning algorithms, and these dangerous events signals will be input into the crisis early warning system. As a result, the corresponding healthcare institution, patient and caregiver will be informed so as to quickly schedule healthcare resources or take any required emergency measures. After confirmation of a crisis, the patient's location will be accurately determined to facilitate the emergency measure treatment. Second, the real-time supervision system receives real-time data such as blood pressure and blood oxygen level values. The virtual model will be repeatedly simulated and evaluated. After iterative optimization, the virtual healthcare model will recommend dosage and frequency of medication according to the EMR system and the PHR data of elderly patients, and will remind the caregiver to monitor the elderly person's health status. Third, the resource scheduling and optimization service will predict which diseases are in high-incidence in each season according to the physical conditions of elderly patients and weather factors. For planning purposes, healthcare equipment and healthcare personnel will be pre-arranged in order to accommodate the peak demands of elderly patients. The cloud healthcare simulation service can help the DTH mechanism to quickly construct simulation scenarios in order to improve the quality and operational efficiency of healthcare services.

4.6 Challenges of Digital Twins

Digital twin technology runs in tandem with IoT and AI technology and hence shares challenges. These challenges should be mapped out first before finding amicable remedies. Several common challenges are found in the IoT as well as data analysis. Challenges in these sub-technologies directly affect digital twin, which should be mapped out for possible solutions. The common challenges are discussed below.

4.6.1 Privacy and Data Security

In digital twin technology, a privacy and data security challenge is obvious due to the robust amount of data used. Some of the data fed to these systems are quite sensitive, and if they fall into the evildoers could lead to financial and other losses. So the system must follow the latest and current updates of security and privacy regulations. Building user trust in these systems is also a significant challenge for digital twin implementation. The end-users should be able to trust their personal information to have confidence in using the system.

4.6.2 Infrastructure

The current information technology infrastructure is a limitation to the demands of the digital twin system. The technology requires information technology infrastructures that would allow for the successful implementation of data analysis and IoT to facilitate effective operations of digital twin. Lack of such infrastructures that are well interconnected becomes an impediment to the implementation of digital twin, making it hard to achieve objectives.

4.6.3 *Data*

The success of a digital twin is dependent on the accuracy and precision of data input. The data should be of high quality, free from noise interference and with a constant and uninterrupted data stream. If the data is inconsistent and inadequate, the digital twin system will underperform and give erroneous output.

4.6.4 *Trust*

Trust is one of the most difficult challenges to mitigate. The digital twin technology ought to be well explained at the foundation stage to make the end-users and the providers understand the benefits, risks and challenges of using the technology. This education aims to overcome the trust issues arising from sharing sensitive data.

4.6.5 *Expectations*

Understanding the population's expectations is a huge advantage and a driving force to digital twin technology. Big technology companies are currently implementing technology, but care should be taken to manage and highlight expectations. The users should understand that digital twin technology is solely meant to solve all the current problems. Both the negative and positive expectations should be well documented to ensure that the appropriate measure is taken when developing digital twin systems.

References

1. Wu C, Zhou Y, Pessôa MVP, Peng Q, Tan R. Conceptual digital twin modeling based on an integrated five-dimensional framework and TRIZ function model[J]. J. Manuf. Syst. 2021;58(B):79–93.
2. Qi Q, Tao F, Hu T, Anwer N, Liu A, Wei Y, Wang L, Nee AYC. Enabling technologies and tools for digital twin[J]. J. Manuf. Syst. 2021;58(B):3–21.
3. He X, Qiu Y, Lai X, Li Z, Shu L, Sun W, Song X. Towards a shape-performance integrated digital twin for lumbar spine analysis[J]. Digit Twin. 2021;1:8.
4. Aubert K, Germaneau A, Rochette M, Ye W, Severyns M, Billot M, Rigoard P, Vendeuvre T. Development of digital twins to optimize trauma surgery and postoperative management. A case study focusing on tibial plateau fracture[J]. Front. Bioeng. Biotechnol. 2021;9:722275.
5. van Houten H. How a virtual heart could save your real one [R/OL]. [2018 11 Dec]. https://www.philips.com/a-w/about/news/archive/blogs/innovation-matters/20181112-how-a-virtual-heart-could-save-your-real-one.html.

6. Chakshu NK, Sazonov I, Nithiarasu P. Towards enabling a cardiovascular digital twin for human systemic circulation using inverse analysis[J]. Biomech Model Mechanobiol. 2021;20(2):449–65.
7. Jung A, Gsell MAF, Augustin CM, Plank G. An integrated workflow for building digital twins of cardiac electromechanics-a multi-fidelity approach for personalising active mechanics[J]. Mathematics(Basel). 2022;10(5):823.
8. Dang J, Lal A, Flurin L, James A, Gajic O, Rabinstein AA. Predictive modeling in neurocritical care using causal artificial intelligence[J]. World J Crit Care Med. 2021;10(4):112–9.
9. Sun T, He X, Song X, Shu L, Li Z. The digital twin in medicine: a key to the future of healthcare?[J]. Front. Medicine(Lausanne). 2022;9:907066.
10. Li X, Lee EJ, Lilja S, Loscalzo J, Schäfer S, Smelik M, Strobl MR, Sysoev O, Wang H, Zhang H, Zhao Y, Gawel DR, Bohle B, Benson M. A dynamic single cell-based framework for digital twins to prioritize disease genes and drug targets[J]. Genome Med. 2022;14(1):48.
11. Baillargeon B, Rebelo N, Fox DD, Taylor RL, Kuhl E. The living heart project: a robust and integrative simulator for human heart function[J]. Eur J Mech A Solids. 2014;48:38–47.
12. Liu Y, Zhang L, Yang Y, Zhou L, Ren L, Wang F, Liu R, Pang Z, Deen MJ. A novel cloud-based framework for the elderly healthcare services using digital twin[J]. IEEE Access. 2019;7:49088–101.

Chapter 5
Cloud, Fog and Edge Computing in 5G

5.1 Introduction

Cloud, fog and edge computing have become widely used computing models to support cost-effective and efficient data processing using commodity servers. Cloud computing makes effective use of distributed environments for tackling large-scale computation problems on vast data set. There are multiple challenges with cloud computing, such as virtualization, isolation, performance, scalability, privacy, and security

Today cloud computing breaks down into three primary form: public cloud where the resources and applications are provided/managed by a third-party off-site provider; private cloud where the data and processes are managed within the organization; and hybrid cloud where both internal and external cloud providers exist. In a public cloud, resources are provided as a service in a virtualized environment, constructed using a pool of shared physical resources, and accessible over the Internet, typically on a pay-as-you-use model. In a private cloud, services and infrastructure are maintained on a private network. Private clouds offer the highest level of security and control. A hybrid cloud comprises both private and public cloud services, which appears to be the best option for many organizations. In Table 5.1, the main benefits and risks associated with each type of clouds are enlisted.

The current computation paradigm has cloud data centers as the only point for execution after the basic processing available at the devices. However, such a large number of IoT devices continuously sending data to the cloud for analysis would lead to scalability issues in the core network. Levels of congestion in the backbone network will increase manifold and may lead to aggravated packet loss and delay, spoiling the user experience. Furthermore, sending lots of data to the cloud for processing may lead to the cloud becoming a bottleneck, again leading to increase in response time. A lot of IoT applications, typically those that run in settings like smart healthcare, need their devices to react very quickly to an impulse. Such a scenario poses the

S. Guo et al., *Advanced Technologies in Healthcare*,
https://doi.org/10.1007/978-981-99-9585-1_5

Table 5.1 Cloud computing: benefits and risks

Cloud type	Benefits	Drawbacks
Public	Low investment in the short run Highly scalable Quicker service to market	Security Privacy and reliability
Private	More control and reliability Higher security Higher performance	Higher cost Must comply with strict regulations
Hybrid	Operation flexibility Scalability Cost-effective	Security, privacy and integrity concerns

requirement of distributed computation, storage and networking services that are close to the source of data, or, in other words, fog computing.

A key element of 5G networks that enables fog computing is small cell (pico- and femtocells), also known as micro-cells. Small cells can alleviate the burden on roof-top base stations (macro-cells) by allowing end points to connect to them. A device can connect either to the macro-cell or to a micro-cell. This makes the architecture of 5G networks a hierarchical one—with the core network (cloud) at the apex, followed by macro-cell base stations and micro-cell base stations, and finally end devices. Hence, from the perspective of fog computing, both macro- and micro-cell base stations form the fog nodes, that is, networking nodes providing computation and storage as well. Packets sent uplink by the devices will be analyzed at the micro-cell or macro-cell base stations before reaching the core network.

In conventional systems, the higher volumes of data will be sent to the cloud, which in turn demands higher bandwidth for transmission of a high volume of data. In addition, the request and response among the cloud and these devices attract higher latency. In order to overcome these limitations, part of the computation can shift from the centralized or cloud systems to the device in the network, which is known as edge computing. This technique results in offloading of workload to the edge from the cloud, which means pushing of computation near to the edge of the network.

Edge computing uses principles of distributed computing, peer-to-peer networking and maybe considered as a natural extension to cloud computing. In edge computing, computing takes place as close as possible to the device in the network, where data are created and require action on data. In addition, it combines intelligence to the data, and this results in the output in the form of analysis, which leverages the AI to provide insights of data in terms of patterns, relations and predictions based on information. As a result, edge computing solution surpasses the benefits of conventional cloud computing and offers several advantages such as real-time data processing, higher performance and building larger echo systems. Edge computing can be summarized by the following equations.

$$\text{Edge Computing} = \left\{ \begin{array}{c} \text{Computing near to the} \\ \text{device in the network} \end{array} \right\} + \{\text{Intelligence}\}$$

Table 5.2 Cloud computing, fog computing and edge computing

	Cloud computing	Fog computing	Edge computing
Data processing location	Process data in cloud data centers	Process data closer to the device	Process data at the edge of the network
Technology focus	Focus on holistic big data processing	Focus on communication issues between infrastructures	More focused on local data processing In addition to focusing on infrastructure, it also focuses on edge devices, placing more emphasis on computing issues
Device performance level	Equipment with the highest performance: large center computer room level	Device performance is low: router, home gateway level	Device performance is medium: base station/ small center computer room level
Advantages	Relatively centralized	Less latency Scalability	Real-time data analysis and intelligent processing Efficient and safe
Relationship	Fog computing can be understood as localized cloud computing, and edge computing is a supplement and optimization to cloud computing		

Table 5.2 outlines the connections and differences among cloud computing, fog computing and edge computing in 5G networks. The rest of this chapter discusses the network architecture of 5G networks and how they will realize cloud, fog and edge computing. In addition, the architecture of cloud, fog and edge applications in smart healthcare is also described.

5.2 Cloud, Fog and Edge Computing Architecture

5.2.1 Cloud Computing Architecture in 5G

Cloud computing can be viewed as a layering architecture, as shown in Fig. 5.1.

The hardware layer includes the physical resources in the cloud, that is, the hosting facilities, servers, switches, routers, hardware middle boxes and power and cooling support. The hardware is typically in the form of data centers, which consist of thousands of servers in racks. The Hardware-as-a-Service provider needs to handle various hardware management issues such as configurations, fault tolerance, backup powers and regular maintenance.

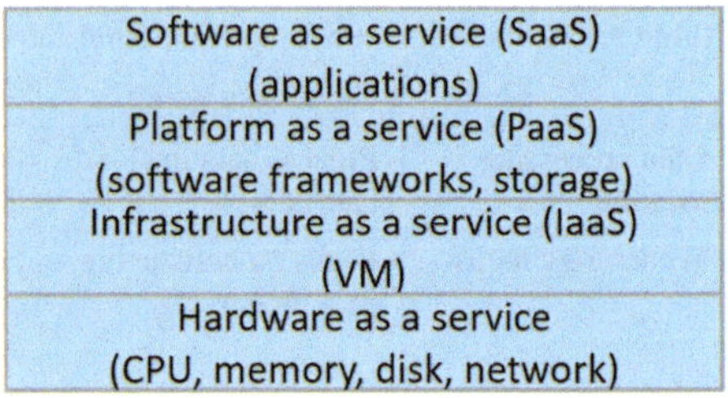

Fig. 5.1 Architecture of 5G network with cloud computing

The infrastructure layer is also known as the virtualization layer. The Infrastructure-as-a-Service provides computing resources as a service. Virtualization is an elegant and transparent way to enable time sharing and resource sharing on the common hardware.

The platform layer includes the operating system and application frameworks (e.g., Java framework) and other system components (e.g., database and file system). Many popular cloud services operate at this level.

The Software-as-a-Service model means that the provider offers software on the common platform as well as the underlying database. Cloud applications can automatically scale as the demand changes.

The layering architecture of cloud computing provides more modular design compared to traditional compute model. Resources are drawn whenever it is needed on demand to fulfill a specific task. Unneeded resources can be relinquished, and the allocated resource is revoked after the task is done.

5.2.2 Fog Computing Architecture in 5G

The architecture of fog network over 5G includes physical network architecture and application architecture. The physical network architecture of a fog network over 5G will extend the architecture of the state-of-the-art heterogeneous cloud radio access networks (HCRANs). The fog network architecture consists of three logical layers that are shown in Fig. 5.2. The devices in each layer are capable of hosting computation and providing storage, hence making it possible for creating complex processing offload policies.

The device layer subsumes all the end devices connected to the fog network. The devices include IoT devices like sensors and also mobile devices like smartphones. These devices may be exchanging data directly with the network or may perform peer-to-peer communication among themselves. Being the source of all data entering the network and the prime actuators performing tasks, these devices are the lowest tier of fog devices. The device layer hosts computation either by embedded coding or as a software running on the operating system of the device.

The fog layer consists of intermediate network devices located between the end devices in the device layer and the cloud layer. The first point of offload in this layer

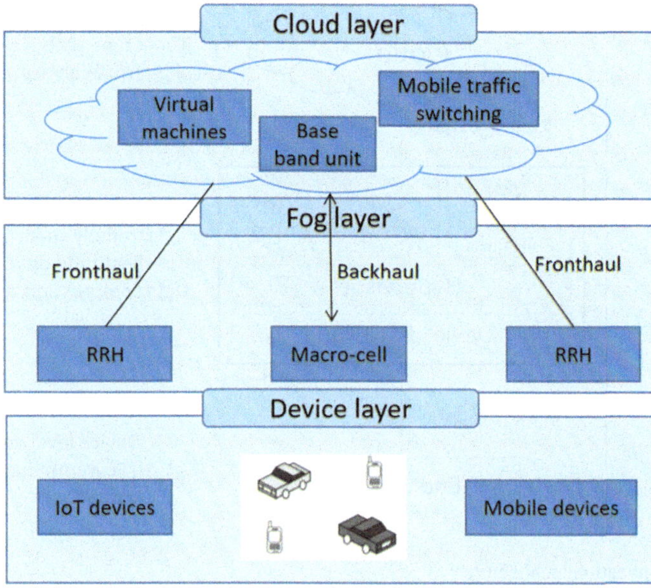

Fig. 5.2 Architecture of 5G network with fog computing—a three-layered architecture

is the remote radio heads (RRHs) and small cells that are connected by fiber fronthaul to the core network. Macro-cells also form a point of offloading processing that send the processed data to the core network through backhaul links. Both fronthaul and backhaul are realized by Ethernet links and the intermediate devices also forming potential places where computation and storage tasks can be offloaded. Each application is packaged in the form of a virtual machine and is launched on the appropriate device. The application virtual machines run alongside the host OS virtual machine over a hypervisor on the fog device.

The cloud layer forms the apex of the hierarchical architecture, with cloud virtual machines being the computation offload points. In addition to application layer processing, the cloud layer contains base band units which process data coming from RRHs and small cells via fronthauls and route processed data to application servers.

An application built for execution on fog infrastructure would have three components—device, fog and cloud components—as shown in Fig. 5.3.

The device component is bound to the end devices. It performs device-level operations, mostly, power management, redundancy elimination and others. Due to the resource constraints of the underlying device, this component should not contain heavy processing tasks.

The fog component of an application performs tasks that are critical in terms of latency and require such processing power that cannot be provided by end devices. Furthermore, the coverage of this component is not global, and this component should host logic that requires only local state information to execute. Depending

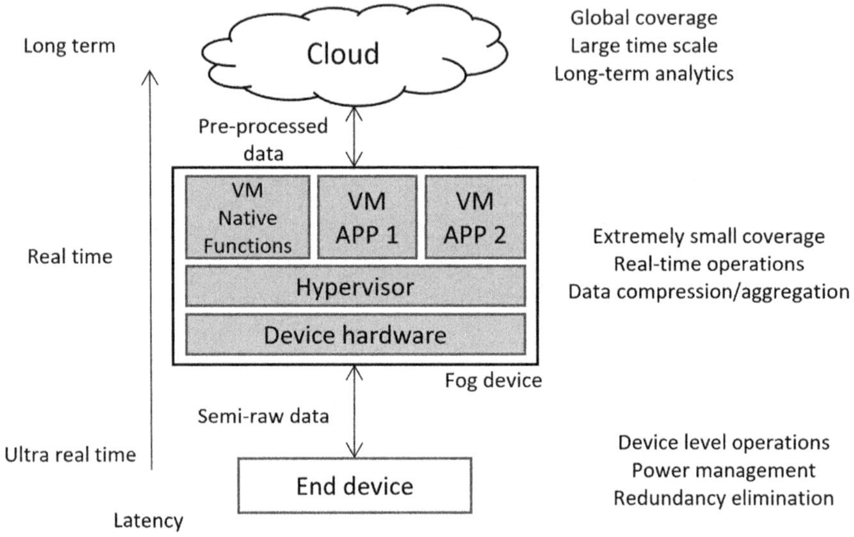

Fig. 5.3 Application architecture

on the geographical coverage and latency requirements of the application, the fog component can be hosted on any of these points of offload.

Cloud component is bounded to the cloud servers in the core network. It contains logic for long-term analysis of the data collected from the lower layers and for operations that do not have any sort of latency constraints per se. Application tasks requiring large processing power and storage are suitable to be placed in the cloud component. Moreover, application logic requiring knowledge of the global state of the system should be placed in the cloud component of the application.

5.2.3 Edge Computing Architecture in 5G

Figure 5.4 shows a typical network architecture of edge network ecosystem that comprises four layers namely cloud, server edge, network edge and device edge. The devices layer comprises of a large number of sensors, controllers and devices actuators. These devices will act as a data source and generate a large volume of data. In addition, the data generated by these devices are processed at the edge of the network in real time. The network layer contains gateways, switches, routers and wireless access points. The server layer consists of edge servers and fog nodes. The cloud layer includes big data processing and handling of business logic. Moreover, a large volume of data is generated, processed at the edge of the devices and sent back to the cloud for storage. Thus, the cloud acts as a data warehouse for the storage of data and provides required intelligence to the edge devices while processing data. To summarize, edge computing architecture facilitates to move execution of applications

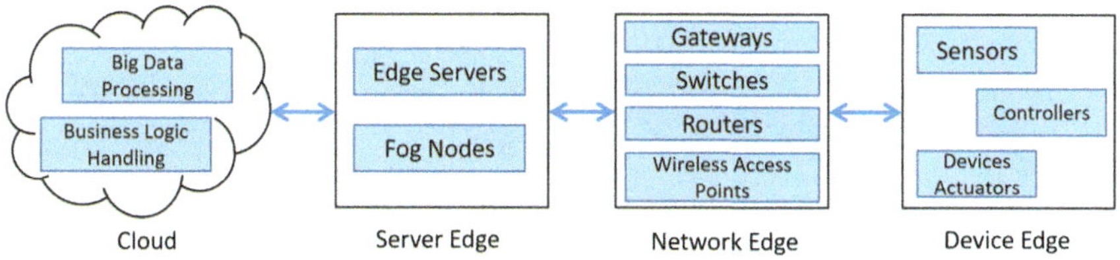

Fig. 5.4 Typical network layered architecture of edge echo system

and data to the edge of the network that is closer to the user, which results in a faster response from the system to the users.

5.3 Application of Cloud, Fog and Edge Computing in Healthcare

5.3.1 Cloud Computing Over 5G in Healthcare [1]

Utilizing cloud computing in healthcare draws enormous interest from the public sector, the research community and industries in recent years. In fact, cloud computing enables healthcare organizations that suffer from a lack of health information technology staff to deploy information technology resources to fulfill various medical demands. Therefore, cloud computing provides excellent value to healthcare organizations and plays a vital role to obtain operational efficiency, staff satisfaction and patient safety in the medical industries.

Cloud computing provides an organized and structured manner to exchange information among patients, caregivers and health professionals, reducing the chance of lost medical data. Figure 5.5 shows an architecture of a healthcare platform based on cloud computing. It has three main layers: the healthcare data analysis layer, the healthcare data annotation layer and the cloud storage and multi-tenant access control layer. The healthcare data analysis layer is in charge of analyzing data stored in the cloud to aid in clinical decision making. In this layer, mining approaches infer clinic routes from individual healthcare records. Then, the patients' healthcare data are compared with historical cases using a similarity calculation module. The healthcare data annotation layer addresses the problem of data heterogeneity that commonly occurs during data processing. The cloud storage and multi-tenant access control layer as a backbone of the platform manages healthcare data collected by sensors' daily activities.

In this section, the application is divided into four main groups, including cloud healthcare services based on data management and risk assessment, cloud healthcare services based on data collection and data gathering, cloud healthcare services based on disease detection and disease prediction and cloud healthcare services security and privacy issues.

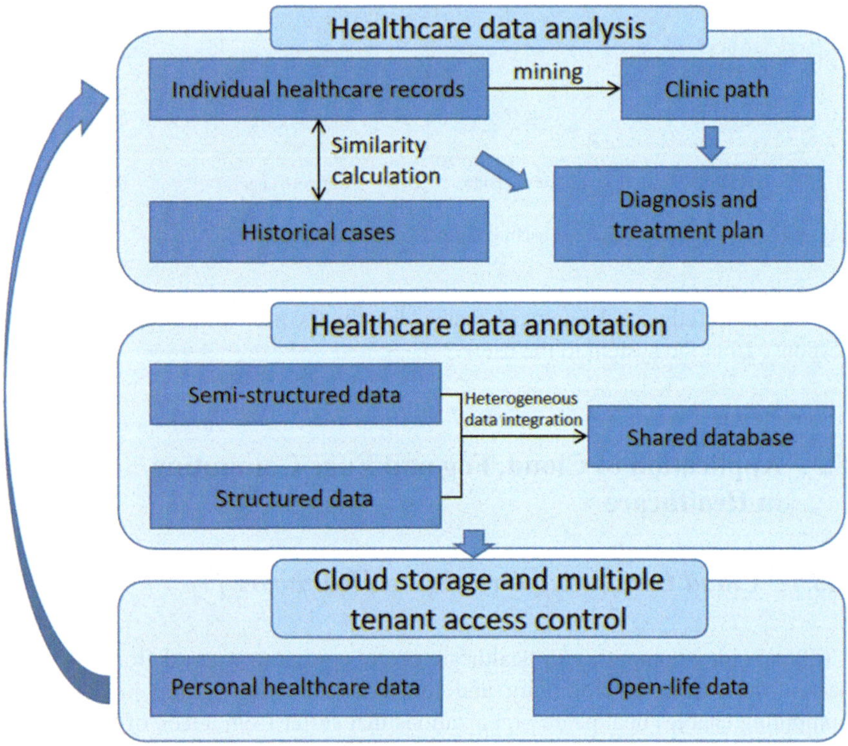

Fig. 5.5 Typical architecture of healthcare platform based on cloud computing

Cloud Healthcare Services Based on Data Management and Risk Assessment. Farid et al. [2] proposed a novel identity management framework for IoT and cloud computing-based personalized healthcare systems. The proposed CloudIoT-based healthcare system has three layers (shown in Fig. 5.6): the device layer, gateway layer and the hospital/public healthcare cloud layer. At the device layer where data acquisition occurs, IoT sensors, wearable devices and other smart devices collect data from patients and send them to the cloud database through the IoT gateway (the gateway layer). The gateway layer consists of a range of networking devices which have access to the Internet. These devices form a local cloud on their own to run the authentication computations. They perform the encryption on the biometric template and save it for authenticating the patient later. The gateway layer also sends the encrypted template to the hospital cloud to ensure that the correct authorization is done in the healthcare database. The hospital cloud layer is also responsible for computing and analyzing the patient's data. This gives rises to several applications that can benefit from accessing this data. It enables healthcare professionals to access the data remotely and empowers other healthcare applications with the capabilities of providing intelligent services such as smart medicine management, emergency alert systems and community-based engagement services.

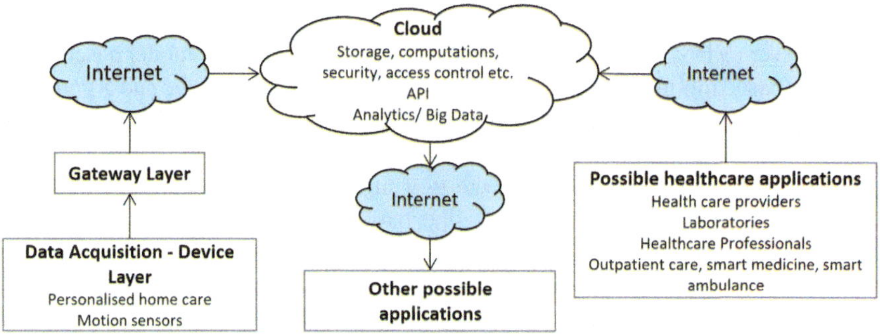

Fig. 5.6 Architecture of CloudIoT personalized healthcare services

Cloud Healthcare Services Based on Data Collection and Data Gathering. Xie et al. [3] presented a fast, robust, learner-efficient and peer-to-peer crucial signal learning mechanism for cloud-oriented healthcare. The overview of the proposed system is shown in Fig. 5.7. The scenario that an elderly patient lives alone at home and his/her physiological conditions are monitored by a remote healthcare system in a medical institution continuously is considered. Various wireless sensors are attached to a patient's body and send the biosignal data to a wearable smart device (e.g., smart watch). The device transmits the data to the private cloud hired by the medical institution for processing. The cloud runs different algorithms for data cleaning, extreme learning machine with semi-model (ELM-SM) training and knowledge discovery. Then the trained ELM-SM is used to measure future clinical states based on newly received data from patients. The clinicians in the medical institution can make diagnostic decisions according to a patient's clinical states and notify the patient properly.

Cloud Healthcare Services Based on Disease Detection and Disease Prediction. The time and cost of chronic illnesses have been reduced with data management using cloud-based healthcare mechanisms. In recent years, designing a comprehensive, real-time and intelligent cloud healthcare mechanism for illness identification and forecasting is more and more popular. Karaca et al. [4] introduced a new mobile

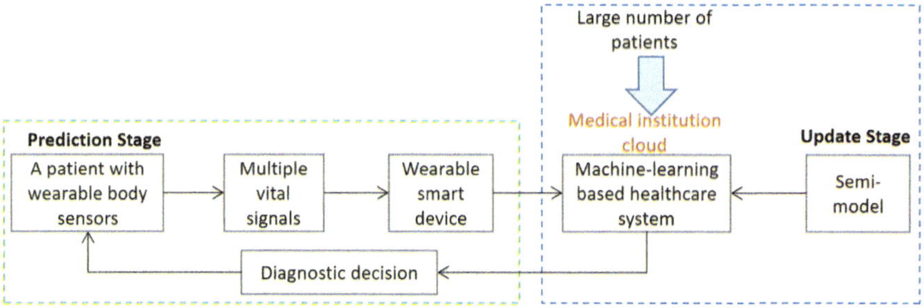

Fig. 5.7 Overview of signal learning system for cloud-based healthcare

cloud computing for the healthcare system for stroke. This study used Virtual Dedicated Server (VDS) as 4 VCPU and 8 GB RAM and proposed a model based on the Android-based mobile phones for stroke patients with cardioembolic and cryptogenic subtypes. The system set up through this study has two basic application elements which are mobile application and server application. Artificial neural network (ANN) module is beneficial for classifying the two stroke subtypes, while server application is used for saving the data from the patients. Zhang et al. [5] proposed an efficient and privacy-preserving disease prediction (PPDP) system in cloud-based e-healthcare mechanism. In their work, patients' historical medical data were encrypted and outsourced to the cloud server, which could be further utilized to train prediction models by using single-layer perceptron learning algorithm in a privacy-preserving way. The risk of diseases for new coming medical data could be computed based on the prediction models. In particular, PPDP was built on new medical data encryption, disease learning and disease prediction algorithms that novelly utilized random matrices. Security analysis indicated that PPDP could offer a required level of privacy protection.

Cloud Healthcare Services Based on Security and Privacy Issues Methods. Security is an important element in the context of information, providing vital and confidential information, for example, in healthcare environments. However, the healthcare system is affected by content privacy and secure data transformation during data gathering and analyzing in cloud environments. To offer a better solution for the above issues, Mubarakali et al. [6] proposed a secure and robust healthcare-based blockchain (SRHB) with attribute-based encryption to transmit the healthcare data securely. The proposed technique collected the data from the patient by using wearable devices in a centralized healthcare system. It observed patient health condition while in sleeping, heartbeat as well as walking distance. The patient obtained data were uploaded and stored in a cloud storage server. The doctor reviewed the patient's clinical test, genetic information and observation report to prescribe the medicine and precaution for a speedy recovery. The proposed method applied to blockchain-based token generation and data security for offering the flexible and compactable privacy of medical records, where the patient health records were collected from a wearable device with a token-based blockchain approach and shared encrypted data for uploading in the cloud server securely. And the doctor would access the patient information after validation of the token-based generated secret key and decryption of health records. Figure 5.8 shows the encryption and decryption process of medical history in a cloud environment.

5.3.2 Fog Computing Over 5G in Healthcare

This section discusses the use case of fog computing over 5G in healthcare and presents a suitable mapping of application logic to application layers for the use case. Distributed system of cameras surveilling an area has garnered a lot of attention in recent years particularly by enabling a broad spectrum of interdisciplinary

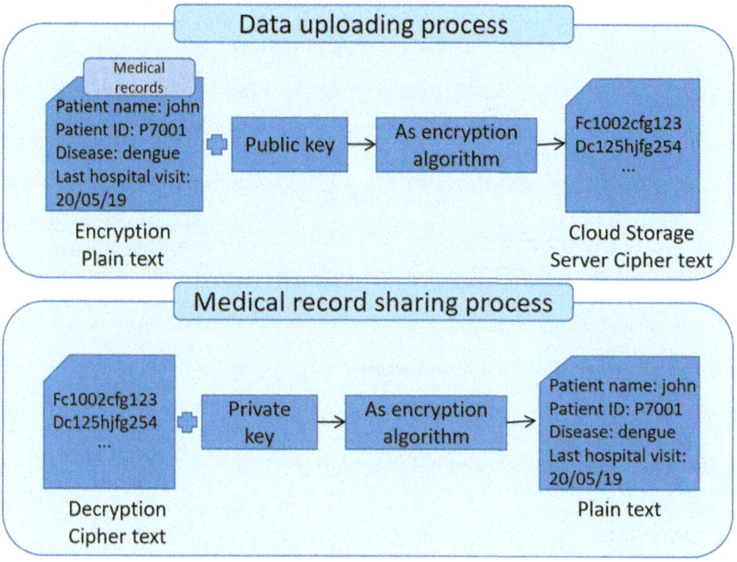

Fig. 5.8 Encryption and decryption process of the medical record in the cloud [6]

applications in areas of the likes of healthcare. Based on the concept presented by Peng et al. [7], a typical deployment of distributed camera analysis system on fog infrastructure is discussed, and it can be applied on smart healthcare in the following. Figure 5.9 shows the necessary components in a smart distributed surveillance system and the interactions between them.

Now, its application architecture for smart healthcare, that is, the placement of application logic into components that can be deployed at different offload points in the fog network, is shown in Fig. 5.10.

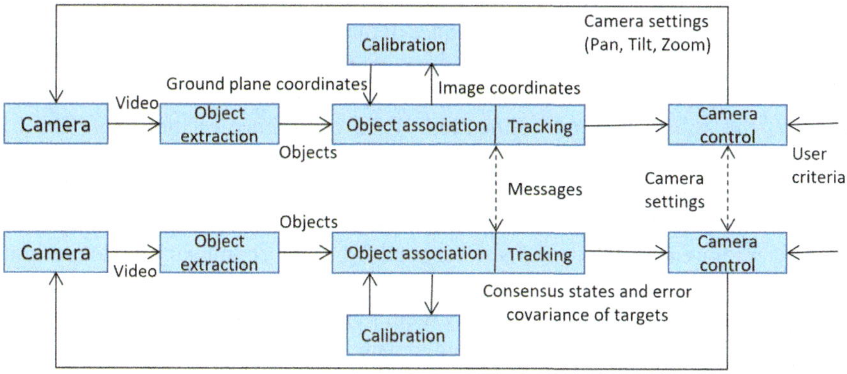

Fig. 5.9 Schematic diagram of a distributed camera analysis system

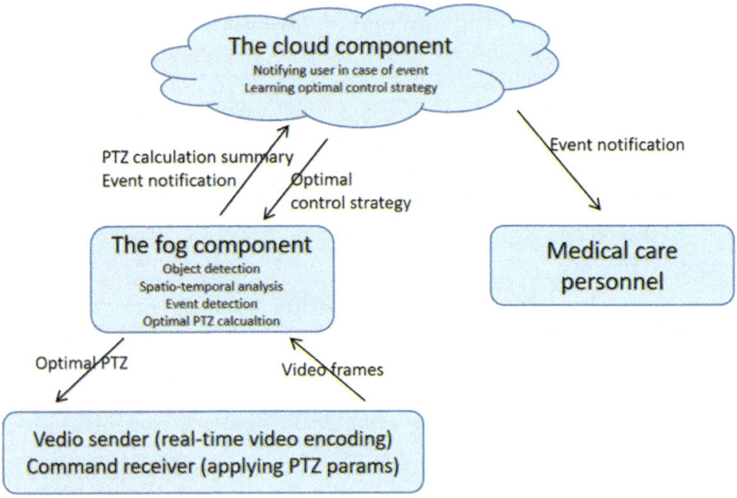

Fig. 5.10 Deployment of a distributed camera network on fog over 5G network

The device component of a distributed camera network application runs on a camera and contains the code for handling it. It essentially consists of two modules—video sender and command receiver. The video sender module sends the recorded frames to the associated small cell at a constant rate. The command receiver module receives instructions to change the camera parameters from the small cell and applies them to get a better coverage of the target. The encoding of video and sending it should take place in real time, as well as the pan-tiltzoom (PTZ) change commands received from small cells should be applied in real time so as to bring down the response time of the data communication network (DCN) to real-time domain.

The fog component of the application is responsible for detecting events based on spatio-temporal relations between objects across video streams coming from different cameras. The application logic first filters out objects of interest from the live camera feeds by using image processing techniques. It then uses the spatio-temporal relations between the detected objects to detect if an event has occurred. In case an event is detected, the fog component informs the cloud component of the application so that users of the system can get notification of the occurrence of the event. The fog component is also responsible for the camera control strategy, that is, tuning the parameters of the cameras in order to optimize the scene acquisition capabilities of the cameras. Based on the camera feeds, the application calculates the optimal PTZ parameters for each camera and also responds to scene complexity by determining the optimal resolution for the camera to capture. These optimal parameters are sent to the cameras in real time which apply them to improve the quality of the captured scene. The fog component sends an aggregate of camera control decisions taken in the past to the cloud component for determining the optimal control strategy, which is then communicated back to the fog component. In a fog setting, placing this component at the very edge, close to the source of data and actuators, greatly cuts down the delay. The only communication between the small cells and the cloud takes place when an object of interest is detected or when the control strategy of the fog component needs to be updated.

The control strategies of cameras can be learned using online learning algorithms. The cloud component can perform the learning based on the information about previous decisions taken by the fog component, use advanced learning tools to determine the optimal control strategy at every time and update the control strategy currently running on the fog component. The cloud component of the application for healthcare enables medical care personnel to monitor the activities in the area surveilled by the DCN via sending notifications pertaining to events of interest to the medical care personnel, who can respond accordingly. In special cases, the cloud component may also stream video related to the event so that medical care personnel may have a look at the actual situation.

5.3.3 Edge Computing Over 5G in Healthcare

In this section, the main applications about edge computing over 5G in healthcare are introduced, including IoT-based automated assisted living care services, disease detection, edge cognitive computing based on smart healthcare system, BodyEdge and multi-access edge computing (EMC) for smart healthcare.

IoT-Based Automated Assisted Living Care (ALC) Services. To assist and monitor people at assisted living care (ALC) is one of the most prominent use cases for edge computing technology in the healthcare domain. Figure 5.11 shows a typical IoT-based assisted living home. An assisted living home is fully equipped with sensors at places near and around to the person. These sensors capture vital signs of the person, including temperature, heartbeat, breathing rate, blood pressure and blood sugar. These sensors act as data source, which are connected to the Internet and transfer data to the nearby edge device. Typically, an edge device may be a gateway. Furthermore, the edge device processes data there itself and then sends it to the cloud environment. A control center is connected to the cloud. Daily activities of the persons and their vitals data are monitored on a continuous basis by a team of medical staff and identified who need the assistance necessary to perform basic activities. Moreover, the staff contacts each person electronically on a daily basis, and these details are recorded. The main advantages of an IoT-based living care centers are the lower number of caretakers, low living costs per person, better control mechanism and paramedical assistance, and the response is nearly real time or even real time. Furthermore, it is easy to extend services such as access to nearby nursing homes, clinical centers, diagnostic centers, hospitals and other advisor services from time to time based on the timely requirements of the assisted living care center.

Disease Detection. Now, numerous machine learning and deep learning algorithms are being used to analyze the data which are collected. To demonstrate how

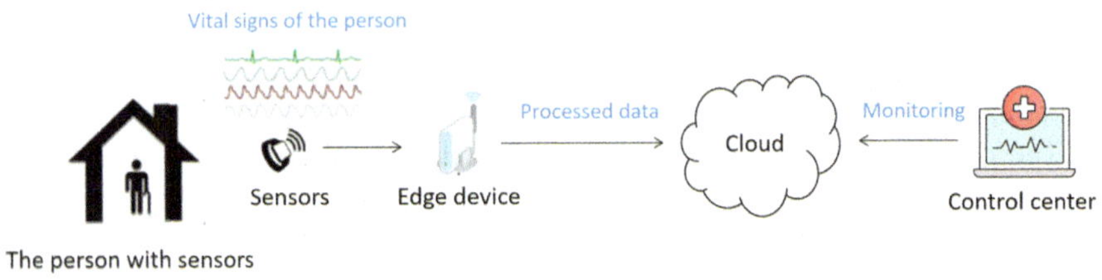

Fig. 5.11 IoT-based typical assisted living home

edge computing can be used along with machine learning and deep learning algorithms in a healthcare system, cardiovascular disease detection has been considered for the case study. The various steps involved in this process have been listed below:

- *Data collection.* A number of devices such as pacemakers, defibrillators and heart rate monitors are being used in order to collect the patient's heart health data, including heartbeat rate, cholesterol level, blood pressure, fasting blood sugar, ECG and so on. The data collected may either be stored on the device or can be sent to the patient's mobile, or even to a personal computer.
- *Data preprocessing.* Since the data are not in a format suitable for performing processing, it needs to be filtered and preprocessed, in such a way that the missing values are handled, categorical data are converted to numerical format, normalized so that the attributes with larger values do not outweigh those with smaller values. After all these steps, data become suitable for the machine learning and analysis.
- *Model creation/choosing a model.* The model may be built using the supervised machine learning or deep learning techniques such as Naive Bayes (NB), decision tree (DT), K-nearest neighbor (KNN), SVM and random forest (RF), or using the unsupervised machine learning techniques such as clustering and neural network (NN). Here, based on the attribute values, it classifies if the patient is suffering from heart disease or not.
- *Model training and model evaluation.* In the evaluation phase, using the methods such as holdout or cross-validation.
- *Make predictions.* The last step is to making the right predictions. The predictions might be image recognition, predictive analysis, semantics or any other kind of prediction.

Based on the case study conducted for the heart disease prediction, the architecture in Fig. 5.12 has been proposed. The data generated by the wearables are collected by the end devices such as mobiles, laptops or tablets. They may be able to process only a small portion of the data based on the computing power available on them. The data will be sent to the edge servers in a wide area network (WAN) for complex computations. Since these edge servers also may sometimes not have all the complex computation required by the data, in such cases, the data will be uploaded to the public cloud for very complex computations and stored on the cloud. The users who may be the hospital staff, research staff or any other can access the processed data from

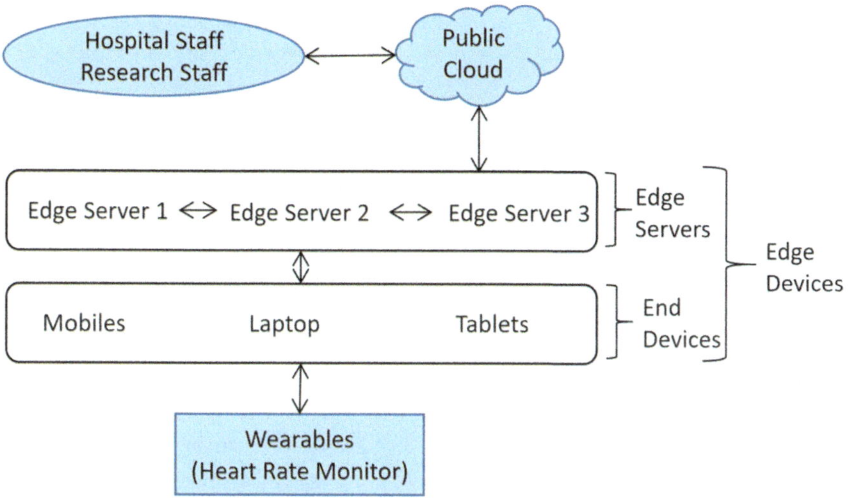

Fig. 5.12 Proposed architecture for edge computing case study on heart disease prediction

the cloud. The complex computations may make use of machine learning or deep learning algorithms based on the application requirements.

Edge Cognitive Computing (ECC) Based on Smart Healthcare System [8]. The ECC-based smart healthcare system leverages data cognition and resource cognition, providing high energy efficiency, low cost and high user Quality of Experience (QoE). Figure 5.13 illustrates an ECC-based smart healthcare system. The data cognitive engine presents the disease risk assessment and gives the priority. According to the basic information, medical history and real-time physiological data of the user, the health risk level of the user is divided into four levels, i.e., low, medium, high and danger. The adopted indexes include age, nature of disease, number of the underlying diseases, respiration, heartbeat, temperature, SpO2 and systolic pressure. The data cognitive engine carries out the comprehensive big data analysis through machine and deep learning on these physiological data of users and transmits the analysis result to the resource cognitive engine, while the resource cognitive engine carries out the resource distribution in accordance with the optimal distribution strategy and feeds back the resource data to the data cognitive engine. Through the static basic information of the users and the disease risk-level information updated by the users in real time, it then combines the dynamic network resource information in the mobile edge computing environment and provides the maximum edge computing resources for the user with the highest disease risk factors. The edge computing environment receives the distribution command of the resource cognitive engine and carries out the resource redistribution of the user side. It can be seen from Fig. 5.13 that in an emergency situation User 4 suffers from a heart attack, and the edge node 2 distributes all the computing resources to User 4 and transfers the other users of User 2 and User 3 to the edge node 1, to realize a dynamic resource distribution. Thus, User 4 can receive sufficient medical service.

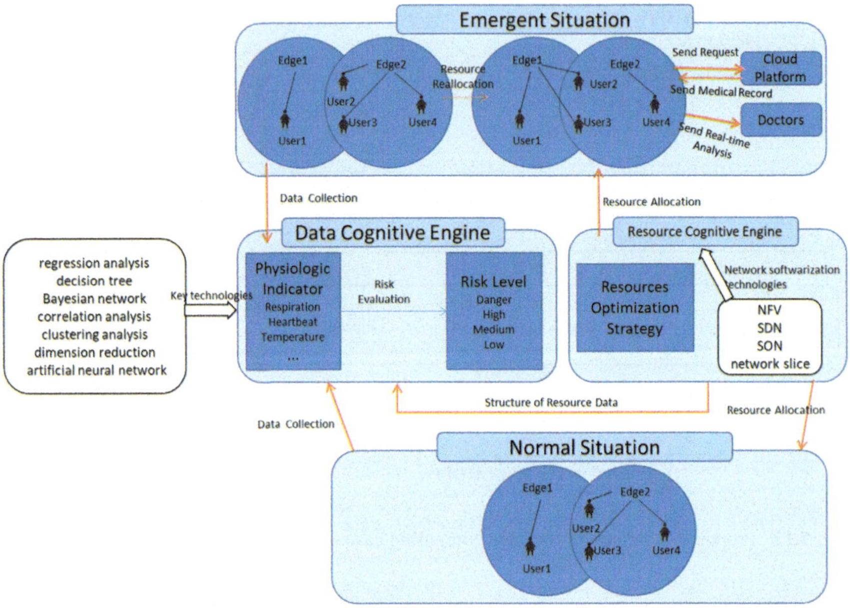

Fig. 5.13 ECC-based smart healthcare system

BodyEdge [9]. BodyEdge is a general IoT system architecture well designed to support specific applications for emerging healthcare industry. It consists of a tiny BodyEdge mobile BodyClient (BE-MBC) software module and a performing BodyEdge gateway (BE-GTW) supporting multi-radio and multi-technology communication to collect and locally process data coming from different scenarios; moreover, it also exploits the facilities available from both private and public cloud platforms to guarantee a high flexibility, robustness and adaptive service level. As shown in Fig. 5.14, the proposed framework is organized in a three-tier (i.e., cloud/edge/IoT devices) architecture in which the edge layer represents the connecting layer between the far cloud and the physical IoT devices whose data can be directly collected from the BE-GTM or through the BE-MBC in specific application contexts.

Multi-access Edge Computing (EMC) for Smart Healthcare [10]. EMC is defined as the ability to process and store data at the edge of the network, that is, in the proximity of the data sources. The advantage of EMC in a smart heath environment is multifold as it can provide short response time, secure transmission and data privacy, decrease energy consumption for battery operated devices and save network bandwidth. The EMC-based smart health system architecture, shown in Fig. 5.15, stretches from the data sources located on or around patients to the service providers. It contains the following major components:

- *Hybrid Sensing Sources.* A combination of sensing devices attached/near to the patients represents the set of data sources, including body area sensor networks,

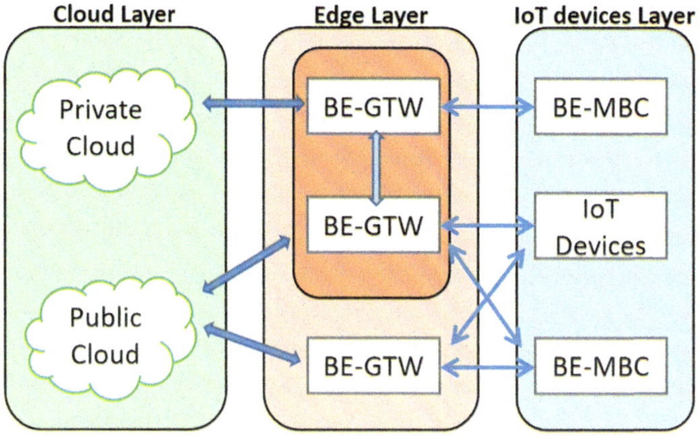

Fig. 5.14 Three-tier architecture of BodyEdge

IP cameras, smartphones and external medical devices. All such devices are leveraged for monitoring patients' state within the smart assisted environment. These hybrid sources of information are attached to a mobile/infrastructure edge node to be locally processed and analyzed before sending it to the cloud.

- *Patient Data Aggregator (PDA).* PDA is working as a communication hub that is deployed near to the patient to transfer the gathered medical data to the infrastructure.
- *Mobile/Infrastructure Edge Node (MEN).* The MEN performs in-network processing on the gathered data, classification and emergency notification, extracts information of interest and forwards the processed data or drew information to the cloud. Importantly, various healthcare-related applications (apps) can be implemented in the MEN, for example, for long-term chronic disease management. Furthermore, with a MEN running specialized context-aware processing, various data sources can be connected and managed easily near the patient, while optimizing data delivery based on the context (i.e., data type, supported application and patient's state) and wireless network conditions.
- *Edge Cloud.* It is a local edge cloud where data storage, sophisticated data analysis methods for pattern detection, trend discovery and population health management can be enabled. An example of the edge cloud can be a hospital, which monitors and records patients' state while providing required help if needed.
- *Monitoring and Services Provider.* A health service provider can be a doctor, an intelligent ambulance or even a patient's relative, who provides preventive, curative, emergent or rehabilitative healthcare services to the patients.

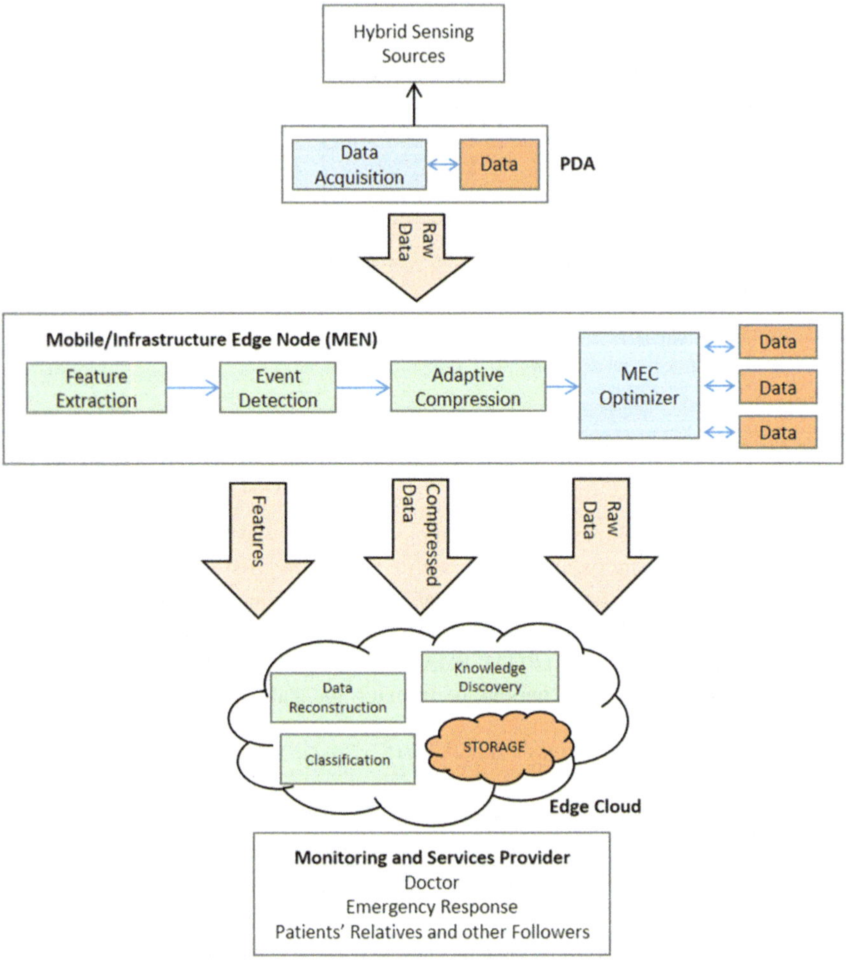

Fig. 5.15 Proposed EMC-based smart health system architecture

5.4 Challenges of Cloud, Fog and Edge Computing in 5G

5.4.1 Challenges of Cloud Computing Over 5G

Cloud computing has gained significant momentum in the past decade. However, it still faces several challenges with regard to performance, security, privacy and interoperability. In the following, the challenges from these aspects are discussed.

Guaranteed performance. Cloud computing dynamically allocates resources on demand, which introduces serious concern on the application aware performance. To provide guaranteed performance, not only the compute resource (e.g., CPU and memory) should be allocated sufficiently, but also the networking resource (e.g., bandwidth and low latency) should be satisfied. The provider needs to have ways to monitor applications' performance so that the service level agreement (SLA) can be met.

Security and privacy. Data integrity and security is a big challenge for cloud platforms, especially for public cloud providers. Encrypting everything in the cloud will introduce additional overhead and may create inconvenience for security monitoring applications.

Fault tolerance. Upon failure, the cloud platform needs to minimize the disruption to the applications and services. Most cloud platform uses seamless migration techniques to restart the application on another physical instance. However, certain infrastructure failures are hard to bypass.

Resource management. One of the most attractive features of cloud computing is the ability to acquire and release resources dynamically as the demand changes. The cloud provider needs automated resource management methods to effectively allocate and relinquish resources while minimizing the operational cost. To achieve that, the operators need tools to accurately monitor the SLAs with low overhead. Mapping the SLAs to low-level resources (CPUs and memory) is itself a challenging problem.

Interoperability. Some applications may need to use public cloud resources when the private cloud's resource is insufficient. Cloud applications may need to run on multiple cloud platforms simultaneously for geographical distribution and performance purposes. All these scenarios require cloud platforms and applications to be interoperable in order to support seamless migration.

5.4.2 Challenges of Fog Computing Over 5G

Fog computing and 5G networks are the enabling technologies for futuristic application in smart healthcare. However, large-scale successful deployment of fog computing systems on 5G networks is bound by research in a number of domains. These challenges are described as follows:

Computation offloading in network base stations. Fog applications run in the form of virtual machines on virtualized fog devices. This would require shifting the network functions—originally implemented in dedicated hardware—to software (a concept called network function virtualization (NFV)). However, implementing NFV on such a heterogeneous network as a fog-enabled 5G network is still not lucid.

Energy efficiency. Fog computing on 5G network requires the base stations to be enabled with virtualization for running applications. Running applications on a hypervisor a higher energy is required due to the heavier processing involved in virtualization. Minimizing energy consumption is a key challenge that needs to be addressed for successful commercialization of fog computing on 5G.

Resource management. Efficient resource provisioning and management has been a strong reason for the success of cloud computing—and will continue to be so for fog computing as well. However, the problem of resource management is even tougher, because of the added dimension of network latency involved. Besides, the vast number of heterogeneous devices in the network further complicates resource management.

Privacy and security. Fog computing virtualizes the network and decouples network functionality from the hardware provider. Hence, fog applications process application data on third-party hardware, which poses strong concerns about visibility of data to the third party. The 5G networks handle voice and data packets in the same manner which may lead to leakage of sensitive voice data. It makes privacy measures even more necessary for fog computing on 5G networks.

5.4.3 Challenges of Edge Computing Over 5G

Edge computing still being in its infancy does not yet have its own framework. In order to design a framework for edge computing, many requirements need to be considered, which bring a new set of challenges as mentioned below:

Programmability. In edge computing scenarios, computation is offloaded from the cloud to the edge nodes. These nodes have different runtimes due to their heterogeneous nature. Hence, when editing an application for deployment in the edge computing paradigm, programmers tend to face a lot of difficulties.

Data abstraction. Data abstraction helps in preparing the data suitable to be uploaded to the cloud. But, it imposes a challenge. When data are trimmed too much, it may cause loss of useful information and, as a result, reduce the precision or accuracy of data. But, when very little data are trimmed, it leads to even the unwanted data being uploaded to the cloud, which can cause extra burden on cloud resources.

Optimization metrics. Edge computing consists of multiple layers, each with different computation capability. This makes allocation of workload in edge computing the biggest issue. When choosing an optimal allocation strategy, it is important to consider the optimization metrics such as energy, bandwidth, latency and cost.

Privacy and security. A home deployed with many IoT devices can reveal a lot of private information through the usage data that are sensed and collected by the devices. In such cases, the challenge is to support the service without harming privacy. When protecting user privacy and data security at the network edge, there exist several challenges including awareness of privacy and security to the community, ownership of data and missing efficient tools.

References

1. Rahimi M, Navimipour NJ, Hosseinzadeh M, Moattar MH, Darwesh A. Cloud healthcare services: a comprehensive and systematic literature review[J]. Trans. Emerg. Telecommun. Technol. 2022;33(7).
2. Farid F, Elkhodr M, Sabrina F, Ahamed F, Gide E. A smart biometric identity management framework for personalised IoT and cloud computing-based healthcare services[J]. Sensors(Basel). 2021;21(2):552.
3. Xie R, Khalil I, Badsha S, Atiquzzaman M. Fast and peer-to-peer vital signal learning system for cloud-based healthcare[J]. Futur Gener Comput Syst. 2018;88:220–33.
4. Karaca Y, Moonis M, Zhang YD, Gezgez C. Mobile cloud computing based stroke healthcare system[J]. Int J Inf Manage. 2019;45:250–61.
5. Zhang C, Zhu L, Xu C, Lu R. PPDP: An efficient and privacy-preserving disease prediction scheme in cloud-based e-Healthcare system[J]. Futur Gener Comput Syst. 2018;79(1):16–25.
6. Mubarakali A. Healthcare services monitoring in cloud using secure and robust healthcare-based blockchain (SRHB) approach[J]. Mob Netw Appl. 2020;25:1330–7.
7. Peng R, Aved AJ, Hua KA. Real-time query processing on live videos in networks of distributed cameras[J]. Int J Interdisc Telecommun Network. 2010;2(1):27–48.
8. Chen M, Li W, Hao Y, Qian Y, Humar I. Edge cognitive computing based smart healthcare system[J]. Futur Gener Comput Syst. 2018;86:403–11.
9. Pace P, Aloi G, Gravina R, Caliciuri G, Fortino G, Liotta A. An edge-based architecture to support efficient applications for healthcare industry 4.0[J]. IEEE Trans. Ind. Inf. 2019;15(1):481–489.
10. Abdellatif AA, Mohamed AM, Chiasserini CF, Tlili M, Erbad A. Edge computing for smart health: context-aware approaches, opportunities, and challenges[J]. IEEE Network. 2019;33(3):196–203.

Chapter 6
Standards Related to Smart Medicine

6.1 Personal Health Device Domain Information Model

6.1.1 Structure Introduction

Personal health device agents all define an object-oriented domain information model (DIM). DIM describes the health device by defining a series of objects. Each object has one or more attributes. Some of these attributes describe the measured health data, and some control or reflect the status of the agent [1]. The model structure is shown in Fig. 6.1.

It can be seen from Fig. 6.1 that the personal health device domain information model uses the unified modeling language (UML) to represent the personal health agent information and class relationship. The top object represents the medical device system (MDS) information and its status. The objects associated with MDS include numerical objects, real-time sampling (RT-SA) sequence objects, enumeration objects, scanner objects or duration measurement storage objects. The duration measurement segment contains the criteria for the duration measurement associated with the duration measurement store. Numeric values, RT-SA and enumerations are derived from a common metric class containing public and shared attributes as a parent class. In general, numerical objects represent situational measurements, RT-SA objects represent continuous samples or waveforms, enumeration objects represent event comments, duration measurement storage, and duration measurement segments can provide continuous storage mechanism for the metrics accessed by the manager subsequently. In addition, scanner objects can help report data transmission initiated by agents.

A series of objects defined in DIM is mainly used to control the agent behavior and reflect the agent's own status update, including the mechanism of measured health data. The DIM of personal health device defines seven objects that can be instantiated. Each object has different functions and concepts. The different combinations of the

S. Guo et al., *Advanced Technologies in Healthcare*,
https://doi.org/10.1007/978-981-99-9585-1_6

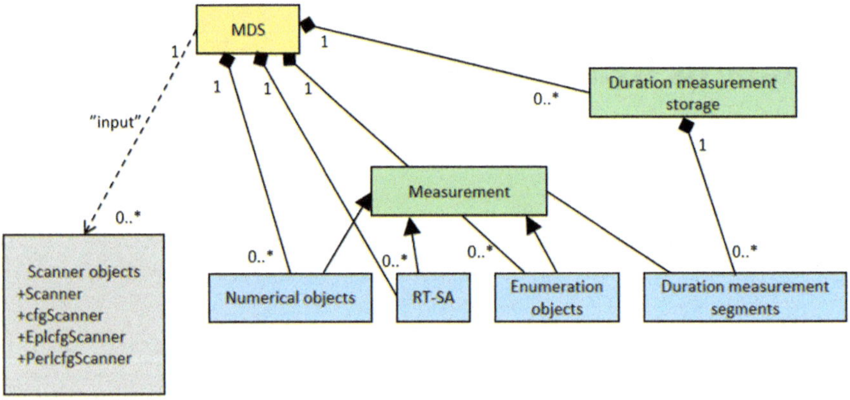

Fig. 6.1 Personal health device DIM

above instantiated objects constitute different configurations of DIM. See Table 6.1 for specific functions and application scenarios.

In the following sections, some examples of personal health device domain information model are given, including the pulse oximeter, the blood pressure detector, the blood glucose meter, etc.

6.1.2 Pulse Oximeter

An example of the hierarchical structure of the pulse oximeter DIM is shown in Fig. 6.2. The MDS class of the pulse oximeter is used as the header of DIM and is responsible for the association and configuration between the agent and the manager [2]. The model includes.

- Numerical objects: blood oxygen saturation, pulse, pulse mass.
- Real-time sampling sequence object: volume diagram.
- Enumeration objects: pulse occurrence, pulse characteristics, device/sensor notification status.
- Duration measurement storage objects: duration measurement storage collects data and duration measurement segment session.
- Scanner objects: cycle configurable scanner and scenario configurable scanner.

The following describes the objects in DIM of the pulse oximeter, as shown in Table 6.2.

Table 6.1 DIM instantiation object

Name	Description
MDS	Each agent has an MDS object, which identifies and reflects the status of the agent and provides other information. Application-specific data (health data) are logically contained in the MDS in the form of information objects
Metric	All base classes representing measurement data, status and context data will not be instantiated by themselves
Numeric	Only one measured value is displayed. Two floating point data types, 16 bytes long and 32 bytes long, are defined through the optimization exchange protocol, which can be a series of numbers or a single value. In addition to numerical value, it can also contain unit and status information. For example, the measurement results of a sphygmomanometer are represented using this object type
RT-SA	The continuous samples or signal waveforms is displayed. The object includes the number of samples and sampling interval. The measurement results of ECG detector are marked by the object type
Enumeration	The status information is displayed in text. The object type includes information such as unqualified product, user's home location or smoke alarm status
Duration measurement storage	Object represents the health database of a large number of measurements stored in the agent. Each duration measurement storage object contains metadata and zero or more duration measurement segment objects. The duration measurement segment contains measured health data
Scanner	The object can observe that the measurement data has been updated and generate an event notifying manager. These events can be events that are regularly reported or warnings triggered by abnormal data. The object will not instantiate itself

6.1.3 Blood Pressure Detector

The blood pressure detector domain information model is shown in Fig. 6.3. The MDS object of the blood pressure detector is used as the head of the model to be responsible for the association between the agent and the manager. The object examples included in the blood pressure detector mainly contain numerical objects, such as systolic blood pressure, diastolic blood pressure, mean arterial pressure, pulse to quantify the numerical factors related to blood pressure, among which the composite numerical objects composed of systolic blood pressure, diastolic blood pressure and mean arterial pressure are mandatory, and pulse value object is optional [3].

The following describes the objects in DIM of the blood pressure detector, as shown in Table 6.3.

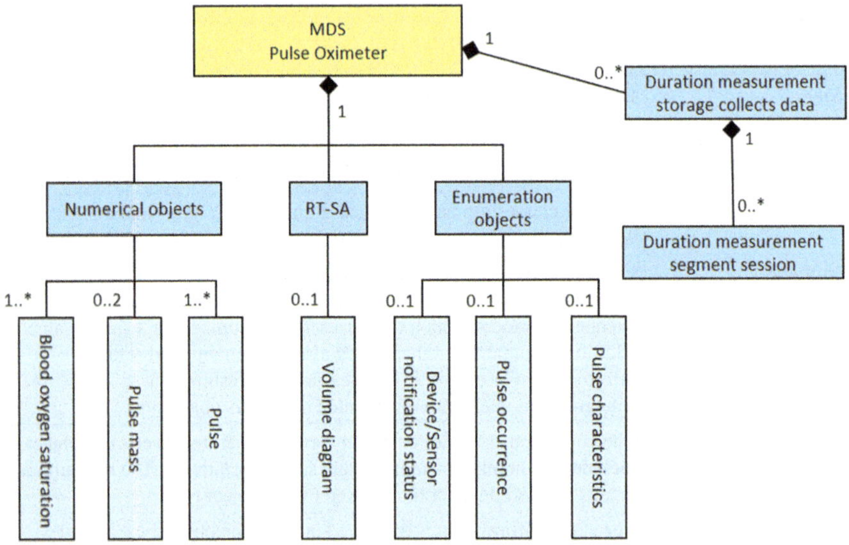

Fig. 6.2 Pulse oximeter DIM

6.1.4 Blood Glucose Meter

The DIM of the blood glucose meter is shown in Fig. 6.4. The blood glucose MDS object is used as the head of the model, responsible for the association between the agent and the manager [4]. The object instances included in the blood glucose meter mainly contain:

- Numerical objects: blood glucose, HbA1c, previous exercise, previous drug treatment, previous carbohydrate, and control resolution.
- Enumeration objects: device and sensor notification status, previous meal, previous sampling location, previous tester, previous health.
- Duration measurement storage objects: duration measurement storage object and duration measurement segment object.

In personal health device, the blood glucose meter is highly portable due to its convenient size, and the user usually carries it with him so that he can measure blood glucose as needed. Therefore, a continuous storage model and a temporary measurement storage model are proposed. The temporary model is to upload the latest data immediately without user intervention, but the storage capacity is small, and the measured values can be uploaded to personal computers or mobile devices frequently. The long-term storage model uploads data according to the request of the manager and applies it to the patient doctor or healthcare personnel. As shown in Table 6.4, each object in the blood glucose meter DIM is introduced.

Table 6.2 Introduction to objects of pulse oximeter

Name	Remark
Standard configuration	The ID assigned to the pulse oximeter device is 0 × 0190 (400) or 0 × 191 (401), which can be used for negotiation and communication during agent and manager association
Extended configuration	The agent determines the objects, attributes and values to be used in the configuration and assigns the configuration identifier (0 × 4000–0 × 7FFF) by itself
Blood oxygen saturation	This numerical object mainly records blood oxygen saturation and related information
Pulse	This numerical object mainly records the properties of pulse measurement
Pulse mass	This object is used to report pulse amplitude information and perfusion volume. It is expressed by multiple methods such as complex average formula and scale factor
Volume diagram	The values in the real-time sampling sequence are intended to represent the plethysmogram, the value of which is the same as the value of pulse amplitude
Pulse occurrence	This enumeration object indicates whether the pulsating event occurs
Pulse characteristics	This enumeration object can convey additional information about pulsating waves
Device/sensor notification status	The objects are enumerated to enable agents to report additional conditions about sensor status, general signal conditions and device status in the device and sensor notification status objects
Duration measurement storage object	This duration measurement storage object stores valid blood oxygen measurement data for several minutes or hours
Cycle configurable scanner	Pulse oximeter can use one or more cycles to configure scanner objects to improve the efficiency of transmitting speed and device information to managers
Scenario configurable scanner	Pulse oximeter can use one or more scenarios to configure scanner objects to improve the efficiency of transmitting speed and device information to managers

6.2 Health and Fitness

Table 6.5 shows several example use cases of IEEE 11,073 series sensors and devices.

A typical user group is composed of healthy people who use various training aids to keep healthy. They use physical health device (PHD) to collect data, store the data in the device, archive data on the personal computer at home and may send data to the fitness coach or personal trainer for evaluation. Users usually own and operate PHD. Users monitor their health status to minimize health problems caused by high blood pressure or high cholesterol or risks caused by family history. They seek the help of professionals to establish and follow the training plan and communicate within the training team. Today, some systems even use data from devices to provide "virtual contests". Users can compare their performance on the Internet. There are many

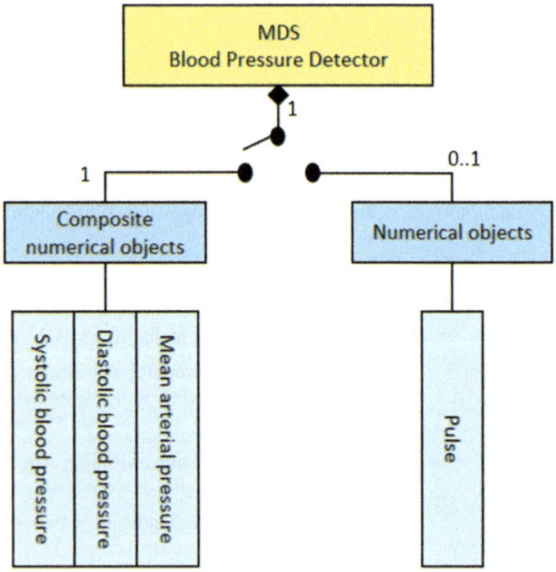

Fig. 6.3 Blood pressure detector DIM

Table 6.3 Introduction to objects of blood pressure detector

Name	Remark
Standard configuration	The ID assigned to the blood pressure detector device is 0 × 02BC (700), which can be used for negotiation and communication during agent and manager association
Extended configuration	The agent determines the objects, attributes and values to be used in the configuration and assigns the configuration identifier (0 × 4000–0 × 7FFF) by itself
MDS	The agent of each blood pressure detector has an MDS object to identify and reflect the agent status and provide other information. Application-specific data (health data) are logically included in this object in the form of information object
Systolic blood pressure Diastolic blood pressure Mean arterial pressure	The blood pressure was measured at different times by cuff sphygmomanometer, and the values of systolic blood pressure, diastolic blood pressure, mean arterial blood pressure and common time stamp were recorded
Pulse	There is a correlation between pulse and blood pressure. This object is used to record the measured value of pulse

other situations, such as the use of PHD by healthy people during pregnancy or in the context of prevention programs.

In reality, typical equipment will not automatically interconnect with systems in other places. Users usually need to actively read the measured values from the

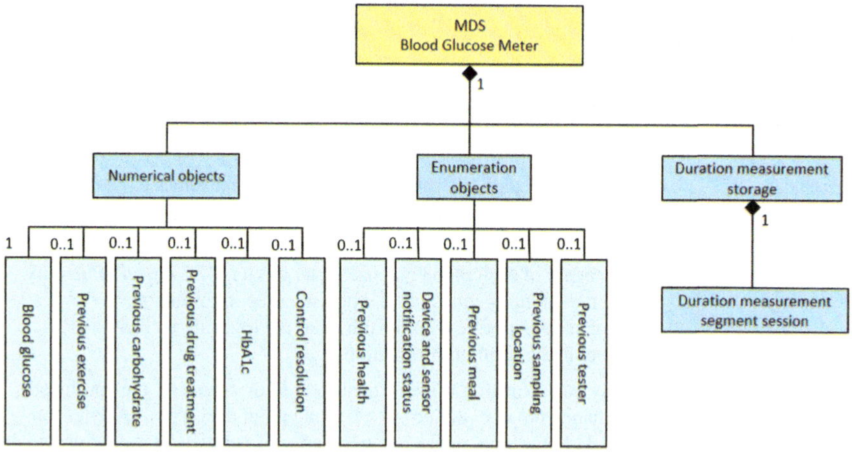

Fig. 6.4 Blood glucose meter DIM

display and input them into the web portal and other types of target systems. In the future, system data from activity sensors and training and intensity data from fitness equipment will be automatically collected. Wireless wrist or body wear devices will be integrated into the clothing to record heart rate, height, speed, calories burned and training duration.

6.3 Disease Management

Table 6.6 shows examples of use cases for disease management and the sensors and personal health devices used.

The typical user population consists of people suffering from chronic health conditions (such as diabetes, chronic obstructive pulmonary disease, heart disease, renal failure and liver failure) and people who have not suffered from the above diseases but face serious health threats (such as overweight, hypertension, hyperglycemia and hyperlipidemia). They use simple personal health devices (such as blood pressure monitoring equipment, blood glucose meter and pulse oximeter) to collect their own data, store them in the device, archive them on personal computers at home and may send them to medical or nursing professionals for evaluation, so as to avoid long-term damage and the development of chronic diseases.

The value of linking these users with professional medical personnel is to reduce the need for face-to-face care with medical service providers, provide care for those in need and reduce unnecessary face-to-face visits. Another benefit is that it can improve the level of treatment and maximize the rehabilitation of patients with chronic diseases. In addition, such preventive health management can improve the

Table 6.4 Introduction to objects of blood glucose meter

Name	Remark
Standard configuration	The ID assigned to the blood glucose meter device is 0 × 06A5 (1701) or 0 × 06A6 (1702), which can be used for negotiation and communication during agent and manager association
Extended configuration	The agent determines the objects, attributes and values to be used in the configuration and assigns the configuration identifier (0 × 4000–0 × 7FFF) by itself
MDS	The agent of each blood glucose meter has an MDS object to identify and reflect the agent status and provide other information. Application-specific data (health data) are logically included in this object in the form of information object
Blood glucose	Only one measured value is displayed. In the standard, the optimized exchange protocol defines two floating point data types, 16 bytes long and 32 bytes long, which can be a series of numbers or a single value. In addition to numerical value, it can also contain unit and status information. The measurement results of the blood glucose meter are represented by the object type
HbA1c	HbA1c, also known as A1c or glycosylated hemoglobin, is used as a long-term measure of blood glucose control. A1c test measures how many A1c hemoglobin cells (specific parts of red blood cells) are saccharified. Since these cells survived for about 4 months, the test showed the degree of blood sugar control in the past few months. This object is used to record the measured value of HbA1c data, calculate value or manually enter value
Previous exercise	The exercise level for a period of time is very important to balance the food intake and insulin dose. If there is a problem of controlling blood sugar, the review of exercise may be helpful to the care and management of people. The object determines the value that a person can enter on the blood glucose device to record his/her exercise
Previous drug treatment	The treatment of diabetes is most effective when the monitoring drug has an impact on the blood sugar level. The ability to track drugs with test results can tell doctors whether a specific drug or combination of drugs is effective. This object is used to record the value of the drug treatment plan of the observation object
Previous carbohydrate	Recording carbohydrate intake is an important auxiliary means for insulin dose management. Although there is a problem of controlling blood sugar, the review of carbohydrates may be helpful for human care and management. This object is used to record the amount of carbohydrate intake, which can directly affect the level of glucose in the blood
Control resolution	The object record controls the resolution measurement
Device and sensor notification status	The device and sensor status notification object allows the recording of specific errors of the glucose meter to track the important troubleshooting information of the manufacturer. The object is described using an enumerated object class

(continued)

Table 6.4 (continued)

Name	Remark
Previous meal	When taking this measurement, blood glucose measurement (or reading) can be further associated with the information of dietary relationship. The test time relative to the meal time can significantly affect the blood glucose level, and this object is described by the enumeration object class
Previous sampling location	Blood glucose measurement can be further characterized by blood sampling location, which is described by enumeration object
Previous tester	The accuracy (or validity) of blood glucose measurement may be affected by the person and place performing the measurement, which is described by enumeration objects
Previous health	Physiological or psychological stress may also be an important factor affecting the change of blood glucose level. This object is described by enumeration
Duration measurement storage	Because of its convenient size, the blood glucose meter is highly portable, and the user usually carries it with him so that he can measure blood glucose as needed. The object supports storing a large amount of blood glucose related data and can avoid automatic deletion
Duration measurement segment	The duration measurement—segmented object included in the duration measurement storage object of the blood glucose meter, which directly stores data measurement values, such as glucose measurement value, glycosylated hemoglobin and health status

Table 6.5 Sample sensors and devices for health and fitness [5]

Domain	Use cases	Sensors and devices
Safe home	Safety of single family life	Independent dynamic field hub, including environmental sensors (such as carbon monoxide)
Life style	Weight management, diet guidance, work-life balance, prevention of burnout, personal health records, online diet diary	Scale, blood pressure monitor, strength fitness equipment, basic electrocardiograph
Physical quality	Cooperative management training, training plan, virtual competition	Scale, basic electrocardiograph, blood pressure monitor, strength fitness equipment
Athletes	Optimize training	Scale, basic electrocardiograph, blood pressure monitor, strength fitness equipment
Family history	Prevention	Blood pressure monitor, drug monitor
Pregnant	Birth	Thermometer, drug monitor, urine analyzer
Prevention plan	Prevention	Scale, activity hub, including environmental sensor and motion sensor, pulse oximeter, drug monitor, peak expiratory flow monitor

Table 6.6 Sensors and personal health devices for disease management

Domain	Use cases	Sensors and devices
Obesity	Monitoring of body weight, medication and treatment	Weighing scale
Hypertension	Blood pressure level management, medication and treatment monitoring	Blood pressure monitor, scale
Diabetes	Blood glucose level management, medication and treatment monitoring	Blood glucose meter, scale
Chronic obstructive pulmonary disease	Monitoring respiratory flow, medication and treatment	Pulse oximeter, peak expiratory flow monitor, spirometer
Heart disease	Remote monitoring of cardiac activity	Blood pressure monitor, scale, pulse oximeter, basic electrocardiogram
Coronary heart disease	Remote monitoring of cardiac activity	Blood pressure monitor, basic electrocardiogram
Heart failure	Remote monitoring of cardiac activity	Blood pressure monitor, scale, basic electrocardiogram
Stroke	Life status, medication and treatment monitoring	Blood glucose meter, blood pressure monitor, scale
Chronic nephrosis	Kidney management	Urine analyzer, thermometer
Liver disease	Liver management	Blood glucose meter, blood pressure monitor, scale

quality of life in the long term and help to avoid the large costs that may be caused in the later stage of professional medical care.

6.3.1 Obesity Management

Development status: Obesity is not only a chronic disease that endangers health, but also an important risk factor for a variety of chronic noninfectious diseases and psychosocial disorders. Personal weight and other data are crucial for users/patients. At present, the treatment of obesity mainly occurs in health centers or medical institutions. The user/patient needs to read the measured value from the scale and manually re-enter it into the target system and use the corresponding application to record the nutrition data every day. The user/patient sends it to the doctor before seeing a doctor, so that the doctor can make the user's daily nutrition plan.

Future prospects: The future obesity management system may automatically collect the user/patient's body weight, body fat content, body mass index and other data through the electronic network scale and other medical and health equipment and transmit these data to the personal computer. Through data heterogeneous transformation, cleaning and analysis, the data that meet the requirements of subsequent obesity analysis are gradually screened out and are calculated for the corresponding body mass index, which will be evaluated by nutrition coaches, trainers or other experts. In addition, this information can be used to develop the user/patient's daily nutrition plan, exercise duration and exercise mode selection. For routine examination or if the expected results are not achieved in time (reduce to the predetermined level), the user may occasionally go to see a doctor. At this time, the summary of information obtained, including daily weight, will be forwarded to the doctor before the visit.

Types of people and roles involved: In addition to users/patients, there are also nutrition coaches, trainers, medical professionals and therapists. Use cases can occur from users' homes to rehabilitation centers, health centers and professional medical institutions.

Reliability, frequency and timeliness of measurement of corresponding PHD: In terms of timeliness, only occasional readings will be taken. If the measurement is lost, there is no immediate risk.

6.3.2 Hypertension

Development status: Hypertension is the most common chronic disease and one of the main risk factors of cardio-cerebrovascular disease. People who work under pressure for a long time have a higher risk of suffering from high blood pressure, and it is difficult for them to arrange regular visits with doctors. At this stage, they can benefit from monitoring blood pressure level and other health conditions to avoid any further health damage or secondary impact on the body. For other people who have experienced serious heart events and need further level monitoring to make them back to healthy, under the guidance of medical professionals, they can also benefit from monitoring blood pressure level, medication and treatment.

Future prospects: Users with hypertension may be equipped with long-term measuring devices, and future hypertension management procedures may use medical and health devices such as sphygmomanometers to monitor users' blood pressure, heart rate or electrocardiogram. The data can be safely transmitted to another system. Through data cleansing, fusion, reduction and other preprocess, the unreasonable data can be corrected, duplicate data can be deleted, image data such as ECG can be multi-scale fused and lossy compressed, and the left ventricular surface voltage of ECG can be extracted for further evaluation by professional medical personnel. Medical professionals help to plan and follow up changes in lifestyle, from adaptive nutrition and exercise plans to rest and recovery stages.

In addition, in the future, the data of all medical devices, including regulated medical devices, can be accessed remotely, and the system status can be tested remotely. At the same time, the future hypertension management service can realize 24-h ECG monitoring and other services. However, online data flow increases the complexity of equipment and requires very high-quality transmission methods and service measures. Therefore, it may not be realized soon. Similar ideas have been put into practice and have achieved good results. Making them more widely used is still a long-term goal with increasing potential.

Types of people and roles involved: The roles involved in this use case are mainly patients who use personal health device, as well as health coaches and medical professionals. The scheme has no regional restrictions.

Reliability, frequency and timeliness of measurement of corresponding PHD: The use case needs the long-term regular measurement, local and online storage, tracking and analysis of trends and display results. Furthermore, the device only occasionally reads data.

6.3.3 Diabetes

Development status: Diabetes is a chronic disease with increasing prevalence. China has become the country with the largest number of diabetes patients in the world. The main harm of diabetes is disability and death caused by chronic complications. At this stage, users/patients with diabetes can be equipped with automatic glucose meters and drug dispensers to record blood glucose levels and drug use. The collected data are usually evaluated by the user/patient first and then by the medical professional. In the networked system, the alarm mechanism is helpful to inform the user and medical professionals of the user's current health status and launch corresponding support activities. In addition, which data are recorded and the interval between measurements should be suitable for each user.

Users with diabetes use subcutaneous sensors to monitor their blood sugar levels, taking readings every 15 min. Users can move freely, go to work, go shopping or participate in professional supervised exercise programs, such as jogging in local parks. Once the blood glucose monitor sends data, it can share information through wireless links to other service providers. The gateway equipment relays the data to the central monitoring station of the local hospital. Users then access data from the central server to obtain their own information, for example, plan meals and adjust drugs accordingly, while the central server sends regular notifications to remind users to inject insulin. This type of system has been demonstrated, and the remote monitoring center operates in many communities around the world, with millions of users and thousands of telemetry reception every month.

In this use case, diabetes often leads to other health problems that need to be addressed. Therefore, a single patient may need multiple monitoring at the same time in a long time.

Future prospects: It is expected that similar systems will become more common in the near future, and remote consultation can be carried out through telephone, e-mail, chat or video conference, and the alarm system of users/patients and doctors can also be included. The long-term vision for the future is to remotely monitor the blood glucose of users/patients and send the control command to the implanted insulin delivery pump according to the blood glucose monitoring situation, so as to optimize the insulin dose based on the current blood glucose reading, analyze and complete the prediction of disease prognosis. The software on the gateway or central monitoring location can display blood glucose information outside the preset threshold window. This allows caregivers at the central monitoring station to contact users/patients and/or dispatch emergency services. In the future, mobile applications based on the standard protocol of personal health devices and the standard information model of personal health records will be developed and evaluated to support effective blood glucose management and standardized services for diabetes patients and assist in blood glucose self-monitoring and medical care for diabetes patients.

Types of people and roles involved: This use case mainly involves users/patients and their medical professionals. This scenario is completely mobile and has no regional restrictions.

Reliability, frequency and timeliness of measurement of corresponding PHD: For internal alarms of parts of interconnected systems, real-time connection is used for alarm. In terms of timeliness, the device takes readings in the important scenarios.

6.3.4 Chronic Obstructive Pulmonary Disease

Development status: Chronic obstructive pulmonary disease (COPD) is still a global health problem, and the monitoring of respiratory flow is one of the important indicators to evaluate lung function. Users/patients with COPD use peak expiratory flow monitor, pulse oximeter and blood pressure monitor to monitor their physical condition. These physical health devices are now available.

Future prospects: The long-term vision for the future is that the next generation of equipment has a standardized interface, and the data can be automatically transmitted to the personal health system at home and sent to the medical remote monitoring service center. Through cleaning, screening and grading of the data and according to the percentage of forced expiratory volume per second (FEV1) in the estimated value, lung function grading will be carried out to help track their health status. The images are used to visualize the changes of users/patients' data, so that medical professionals in the service center can view the change trend of the incoming data and automatically notify users/patients. Healthcare professionals can contact users/patients to discuss their symptoms, suggest lifestyle changes or ask them to arrange a visit for other diagnosis.

Types of people and roles involved: Like diabetes management, this use case mainly involves users/patients and their medical professionals. The scenario is completely mobile and has no regional restrictions.

Reliability, frequency and timeliness of measurement of corresponding PHD: For internal alarms of parts of interconnected systems, real-time connection is used for alarm. In terms of timeliness, the device takes readings in the important scenarios.

6.3.5 Heart Disease

Development status: At present, the overall number of patients with heart disease is increasing, which leads to more and more research on the prevention and treatment of heart disease. Special ambulatory ECG device (e.g., Holter monitor) is designed to continuously monitor the electrophysiological status of human heart for at least 24 h. Its extended recording time can sometimes be used to observe sporadic arrhythmia that is difficult to recognize in a short time. At this stage, Holter monitors record the cardiac electrical signals obtained through electrodes connected to the body during the whole recording period, and networked monitors can transmit data in real time at the end of the recording period. Some devices available at present provide these types of interfaces, but most of them are not standardized.

Future prospects: The application of future records to realize end-to-end standardized data connection will help to transmit monitoring data to professional medical service providers, detect and process abnormal data such as wrong data, invalid data, duplicate data through data heterogeneous transformation, cleaning and analysis, verify the correlation of the data, mine disease correlation, and screen out abnormal cardiac electrical signals. The process of heart disease association analysis is visualized in the form of images to support patient care in a broader range.

Types of people and roles involved: This use case mainly involves users/patients and their medical professionals. The scenario is completely mobile and has no regional restrictions.

Reliability, frequency and timeliness of measurement of corresponding PHD: The use case needs the long-term regular measurement, local and online storage, tracking and analysis of trends and display results.

6.4 Home Health Monitoring

Table 6.7 shows the home health monitoring use cases and sample sensors and devices used.

Various sensors and devices are needed at home, as shown in the following examples, which can remind users to help themselves, for example, taking drugs. If the user's behavior or health condition changes suddenly and potentially, they will remind others, such as relatives and nearby care providers. The fall sensor installed on the body can notify the monitoring system of a potential fall event. In order to improve the safety of the home, users use Personal Emergency Response Sensor (PERS) to call others for help. It is usually in the form of pressing a button to indicate an emergency.

For the elderly who live alone, the sensors that monitor life health can be combined with other sensors that perceive the family environment. Future families will provide devices for collecting and interpreting data from all available sources, such as providing and distributing data through home networks and promoting the sharing of

Table 6.7 Sensors and personal health devices for home health monitoring

Domain	Use cases	Sensors and devices
Home care	Prevention	Independent on-site dynamic hub, drug monitor, blood pressure monitor, scale, thermometer
Congenital disorder	Monitoring	Independent on-site dynamic hub, drug monitor, blood pressure monitor, scale, thermometer, pulse oximeter, basic electrocardiograph
Geriatric care	Accident prevention, monitoring	Independent on-site dynamic hub, drug monitor, blood pressure monitor, scale, thermometer, blood glucose meter, pulse oximeter, basic electrocardiograph
Recovery	Monitoring, speed up the rehabilitation process	Independent on-site dynamic hub, drug monitor, blood pressure monitor, scale, thermometer, blood glucose meter, pulse oximeter, basic electrocardiograph

this information with doctors and relatives through the Internet. Sharing data between these different systems requires a common set of standards. With the increase in the number of elderly people with chronic diseases, a home medical set-top box (connected with electronic scales, sphygmomanometers and blood glucose meters) can be installed as a chronic disease management center to manage their chronic diseases. It can collect health data according to PHD standards and provide chronic disease care services according to the collected data. Table 6.8 shows the physical requirements of elderly patients at home for data transmission.

Types of people and roles involved: Participants in this use case are friends and relatives, therapists and medical professionals. The typical scenario is family, but it may extend to mobile environment.

Reliability, frequency and timeliness of measurement of corresponding PHD: As for independent living, it is very important to receive real-time readings of drop

Table 6.8 Physical requirements for data transportation of household medical equipment for the elderly

Device	Data category	Transmission rate (ms)	Application layer throughput (kb/s)	Maximum end-to-end delay	Minimum range (m) or coverage area (m^2)
Bed sensor	Location status change (real time)	8	0.02	15 min	15 m, 2 m^2
Drop detector	Position alarm (real time)	8	0.02	15 min	15 m
Pill dispenser	Remind	200	0.02	60 min	15 m, 2 m^2
Visual telephone	Video/audio	On demand	384	300 ms	4.5 m, 15.75 m^2

sensors in time. If the equipment fails and the data are lost or damaged, a major risk will occur. These need to be properly addressed.

References

1. Health informatics—personal health device communication—part 20601: application profile—optimized exchange protocol: ISO/IEEE 11073-20601:2016 [S/OL]. [2016 June 15]. https://www.iso.org/standard/66717.htm.
2. Health informatics—personal health device communication—part 10404: device specialization—pulse oximeter: ISO/IEEE 11073-10404:2010 [S/OL]. [2010 May 01]. https://www.iso.org/standard/54572.html.
3. Health informatics—personal health device communication—part 10407: device specialization—blood pressure monitor: ISO/IEEE 11073-10407:2010 [S/OL]. [2010 May 01]. https://www.iso.org/standard/54573.html.
4. Health informatics—personal health device communication—part 10417: device specialization—glucose meter: ISO/IEEE 11073-10417:2010 [S/OL]. [2010 April 19]. https://www.iso.org/standard/70739.html.
5. Health informatics—personal health device communication—part 00103: overview: ISO/IEEE 11073-00103:2015 [S/OL]. [2015 March 01]. https://www.iso.org/standard/64941.html.

SPRINGER NATURE

GPSR Compliance

The European Union's (EU) General Product Safety Regulation (GPSR) is a set of rules that requires consumer products to be safe and our obligations to ensure this.

If you have any concerns about our products, you can contact us on ProductSafety@springernature.com

In case Publisher is established outside the EU, the EU authorized representative is:

Springer Nature Customer Service Center GmbH
Europaplatz 3
69115 Heidelberg, Germany

The manufacturer's authorised representative in the EU is Springer Nature Customer Service Centre GmbH, Europaplatz 3, 69115 Heidelberg, Germany. If you have any concerns regarding our products, please contact ProductSafety@springernature.com

Printed and bound by CPI Group (UK) Ltd, Croydon, CR0 4YY
01/10/2026
02225919-0014